Praise for Inside-Out Health

Dr. Robert Silverman's book is a magnificent tour de force full of practical tips on how to use functional medicine to stay fit and healthy and lose weight, starting with the gut. If you are frustrated with your health, wanting to rid yourself of body pains, and looking for ways to achieve total wellness, Inside-Out Health is a great start to a happy gut and overall well-being!

— Vincent Pedre, MD, author of *Happy Gut: The Cleansing Program to Help You Lose Weight, Gain Energy, and Eliminate Pain*; founder of Dr. Pedre Wellness

Many of us have lost our way when it comes to our body. We ignore our instincts and inherent ability to know what we need to heal. Dr. Silverman gives us Inside-Out Health to reset our connection to our inner self and navigate our way back to our innate intelligence of the what, how, and why of health and healing.

— Deanna Minich, PhD, functional nutritionist and author of *Whole Detox*

I credit Dr. Silverman for a lot of my physical health—he's taken a chance on me when other doctors wouldn't. He's really helped relieve the stress and pain that playing ball in the NBA can cause. Doctors like Dr. Silverman are hard to find. If you can't see him in person, read his book instead!

– Sean Kilpatrick, NBA shooting guard

This book is just what the doctor ordered. Dr. Robert Silverman takes the reader on a healing journey using his revolutionary "inside-out" approach. Starting with the gut microbiome and leaky gut syndrome (a topic foreign to the majority of medical doctors), Dr. Rob guides us on the causes and solutions to most medical ailments. The book is easy to read and packed full of practical health tips. A must-read for any health enthusiast and physician looking to understand how the body really works.

– Jack Wolfson, DO, FACC, author of *The Paleo Cardiologist*

Dr. Rob Silverman has written an excellent book looking at health and nutrition from a new perspective. In easy-to-understand language, he explains important concepts such as how to create a healthy environment for good gut bacteria. He clearly lays out his six-step plan for helping you heal your gut. In other chapters, he discusses weight issues, concussions, the use of laser therapy, and other important healing topics.

Inside-Out Health is well written and full of helpful hints, regardless of your age or medical history.

– Thomas E. Hyde, DC, DACBSP, FRCCSS (Hon), author and editor of *Conservative Management of Sports Injuries*

Dr. Rob Silverman has been a leader in the field of integrative and holistic medicine for over fifteen years! Now he is able to share his knowledge beyond the office setting. In Inside-Out Health, Dr. Silverman has turned the health-care paradigm upside down. A must-read for understanding the root causes of illness as well as a return to healthy living. Dr. Silverman gives us a step-by-step overview of all the major systems that govern our well-being, from the broad picture down to the minor details. In reading his book, you will experience real and sustainable changes to your life.

– Christopher Keroack, MD, IFMCP, author of *Changing Directions: Navigating the Path to Optimal Health and Balanced Living*

Dr. Silverman's book Inside-Out Health is a must-read for individuals wanting to take their health and bodies to another level. It gives the reader a broad range of treatment options and lifestyle changes that could prove to be life-saving. Being a professional racecar driver puts a lot of stress on your body, especially when you add Crohn's disease into the mix. The extreme temperatures and physical loads can take a toll on your health, not to mention the constant traveling and training to prepare for races. Dr. Silverman took the time to understand my issues and helped me adjust my lifestyle health plan. I'm symptom-free, sleeping great, and digesting food properly. I now have the energy levels I need to push myself in the gym and on the track. Most importantly, I'm driving better than ever!

– W. Lawson Aschenbach, professional racecar driver, multi-time champion, diagnosed with Crohn's disease

As an avid reader of clinical health books, I was captivated with Dr. Silverman's new book Inside-Out Health. He gracefully and in plain English explains how to obtain better health through his time-tested Six R gut program. Dr. Silverman pulls the curtain back on new scientific discoveries on toxins and obesity. This alone may be worth the cost of the book. His detailed review of inflammation and its relationship to the root cause of almost every health issue is sure to make you sit up and realize that this can change your life in a major way. I applaud Dr. Silverman for sharing his passion and love to help sick people get well.

– Ron Grisanti, DC, DABCO, DACBN, MS, medical director of Functional Medicine University

The body has a tremendous ability to heal itself from inside out. The vast majority of medical approaches in our healthcare system are directed at treating symptoms from the outside in. Dr. Silverman takes his entertaining, vibrant teaching skills and explains how to take charge of your own health. Dr. Silverman gives you the tools you need to allow your body to live its life to the fullest expression. Following the guidelines and protocols he describes in this must-read will add years to your life and life to those years.

— Scott J. Banks, DC, Institute for Functional Medicine Certified Practitioner; author of *Natural Cures for Dummies*

I've met many great clinicians in my career, and I've also met many great academics. Dr. Robert Silverman is one of those rare individuals who is both. He can thoroughly explain the scientific understanding and also put the clinical application into practice. Success in every aspect of practice is tied directly to the outcomes we get with our patients. There is no way you can read this book without becoming a better, more competent doctor.

— Dane Donohue, DC, creator of 8 Weeks to Wellness; author of *Fat, Fatigued and Fed Up*

Medicine should heal from the inside out. Dr. Silverman has excelled in delivering this message through a thoughtful approach to applying functional nutrition. This is core healing at its best, applicable to all chronic disease. It is a book everyone should read!

– Alison Monette, ND, RD, national speaker

Dr. Silverman is a chiropractor's chiropractor. The information in this book is priceless if you want to live a long, healthy, and active life. Read this book to learn the fundamentals on how to get and stay healthy. Health is an investment in your future—start today by reading this book!

– Brad Weiss, DC, Performance Health Center

Dr. Rob Silverman is a nutrition expert and a chiropractor's chiropractor. In Inside-Out Health he shares current science and actionable steps for choosing your nutrition wisely to reduce inflammation and regain your health. Dr. Silverman's outside-the-box answers for chronic health problems help his patients return to vitality and enjoy life through nutrition and physical activity. His solutions work!

– Steven Weiniger, DC, Posture Expert, BodyZone.com

INSIDE-OUT HEALTH

Inside-Out
HEALTH

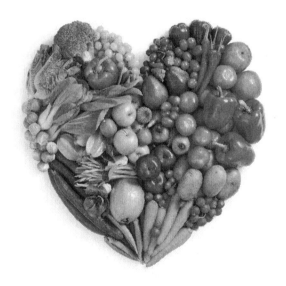

A Revolutionary
Approach to Your Body

DR. ROBERT G. SILVERMAN

INSIDE-OUT HEALTH

A Revolutionary Approach to Your Body

ISBN   978-1-61961-448-2 *Hardcover*
       978-1-61961-449-9 *Paperback*
       978-1-61961-450-5 *Ebook*

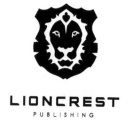

LIONCREST
PUBLISHING

For my wife MeiMei, whose loving support and patience with my long days and late nights makes all the difference. And for my parents, Lloyd and Isabel, who raised me to work hard, care for others, and always do my best. My success is theirs.

Contents

Introduction

A New View

Treat the system, not the symptom.

People today are getting sicker, not healthier. We don't have a health-care system—we have a sick-care system. 133 million Americans have a chronic disease or condition. The annual cost of chronic pain is as high as $635 billion a year. That's more than the annual costs for cancer or heart disease.

Nearly 35 percent of the American population is overweight or obese. We're not the only ones; around the world, people are following our leadership by getting heavier. Currently, nearly 30 million Americans have type 2 diabetes; of those, about 8 million have it but don't know it yet. By 2030, researchers estimate that half of all Americans will have either prediabetes or type 2 diabetes. It's time for a new view.

Many of us approach our health backward, focusing on the effects rather than the causes, and focusing on symptoms instead of systems. That's the way conventional medicine looks at treatment. In functional medicine and nutrition, we take a different approach. We look at the symptoms, but then we look upstream in the body's systems to see where the real cause of the problem lies.

In 1985, the government allowed drug companies to advertise their products directly to consumers. Since then, we've had Pharmageddon—an epidemic of overmedication.

THE BACKWARD APPROACH TO HEALTH CARE

As a functional chiropractor and nutritionist, when I see a symptom, I know that something is wrong with the system. The traditional medical approach is to treat the symptom. The functional approach is to treat the system. The medical approach usually involves drugs that work quickly by shutting off the pathways that are causing the problem. A good example would be drugs to reduce stomach acid, which work by turning off the mechanism that makes the acid. As it turns out, however, these drugs sharply increase the risk of kidney disease in people who use them over the long term. The functional approach to excess stomach acid might be short-term use of an acid-blocking drug while we figure out the upstream cause and ways to modulate the pathways, not switch them off. That usually involves therapeutic lifestyle changes and nondrug approaches that take longer to work. There are certainly times, such as a bad infection, when the quick, brute-force approach of powerful drugs is absolutely the right thing to do. But in my experience, the dramatic, long-lasting improvements don't come from drugs; they come from within as a patient makes lifestyle changes.

DR. ROBISM

Nutrition is like shoes. There's no "one size fits all."

INSIDE-OUT HEALTH

DR. ROBISM

Beauty is only skin deep, but health runs deep throughout the body.

We spend a lot of time worrying about how we look on the outside, when what we should really worry about is what's on the inside. Beauty really is only skin deep.

Nobody ever thinks about how having a beautiful liver is a lot better than having high cheekbones, but it is. (I'll explain that more in Chapter 3 on detoxification.)

In this book, I'll be challenging the conventional protocols for treating almost all common health issues. I'll be recommending treatments such as detoxification that work from the inside out to treat the underlying cause of many health concerns. I take the functional approach, which is to look upstream within the body for the cause of downstream problems. I use functional nutrition to help the body's own pathways heal with a little help. As I like to tell my patients, you can see the trunk, branches, and leaves of a tree, but there's just as much of a tree underground as above ground. When you see a tree, you see leaves. The leaves are the symptom, the tree is the external system, and the roots are the internal system. No system is one-way or completely separate from every other system in your body.

THE MUSCULOSKELETAL SYSTEM

Back pain is a $765 billion industry that relies largely on dangerous pain-killing drugs and treatment modalities that don't help. Eight out of ten people will have at least one episode of severe lower back pain in their lifetime. Half of all back surgeries fail.

As a chiropractor, I know that chiropractic therapies can help back pain—and we have a lot of very solid research to prove it. I also know that truly treating back pain, so that it goes away and doesn't come back, doesn't need drugs, physical therapy, and surgery. It needs an inside-out approach. As I'll explain in Chapter 4, we need to treat the chronic inflammation that underlies a lot of musculoskeletal problems. We also need to help the patient lose weight, detoxify the body, restore a healthy balance of gut bacteria, learn how to strengthen the core muscles, and move better (see Chapters 5 and 6 for that).

How do your gut bacteria connect with your muscles? I'll explain this in detail in Chapter 4. For now, let's just say that you have trillions of bacteria living in your gut. In fact, you have more bacteria in your gut than you have cells in your body. You're basically just a super organism supporting a very large colony of bacteria. You may think you're in charge, but you're not—your bacteria are. When your bacteria aren't happy because they're out of balance and not getting the right nutrients from your diet, you get inflamed. Inflammation causes joint and muscle pain, damages the connective tissue, and slows healing of injuries. Get your bacteria into a healthy balance, and a lot of inflammation disappears and takes the joint and muscle pain with it. This is a really good example of inside-out health. Instead of tackling the inflammation with powerful anti-inflammatory drugs, you tackle it by reducing your inflammation from within.

WORKING WITH ME

The functional approach to health puts a lot of responsibility on the patient. You can't just pop a pill; you need to be proactive in your treatment and have the patience to see it through. When you work with me, I'm your teacher and your coach. No coach has a perfect record, but if you don't do well, I bear the blame. I need you to tell me what it will take to get you to do what you have to do and stay with it. I'll do whatever it takes, because my goal in life is to help people. My reward is to see you really understand why you need to make the changes, do it, internalize it, get better, and stay better.

WHAT YOU'LL LEARN

In this book you'll learn about inside-out treatments for the most common conditions, the things that patients come to me for the most.

In Chapter 1, you'll learn all about your gut and the bacteria that live there. In particular, you'll learn about leaky gut syndrome, a very common but frequently undiagnosed problem that is best treated from the inside out.

Chapter 2 is where you'll learn about bone and joint health and why the usual treatments for arthritis are completely backward. You'll discover how inflammation can be both helpful and harmful and how you can change the balance from the inside out.

The role of toxins in harming our health is what Chapter 3 is all about. Accumulated environmental toxins in the body are a major underlying cause of health problems. In this chapter you'll learn why detoxing your body helps you heal from the inside out.

In Chapter 4, you'll gain a full understanding of our current epidemic of inflammation and how it's at the root of almost every health issue. You'll learn how to turn down your inflammation from the inside.

Chapter 5 deals with our fast-growing obesity epidemic. You'll learn why diets don't work and why I never recommend them for my patients. You'll also learn what inside-out approaches do work for weight loss.

Life is motion, a concept I'll discuss in detail in Chapter 6. Here you'll learn how to strengthen the all-important core muscles to keep you standing strong and straight.

I'm not a huge fan of using every new technology that comes along, but lasers are different. As you'll learn in Chapter 7, they heal from the inside out.

Chapter 8 discusses soft-tissue injuries. These common problems can be painful and even disabling—but they can also be very responsive to inside-out approaches.

Awareness of concussion has sharply increased recently. As I'll explain in Chapter 9, that's an important step in the right direction for treating these serious injuries. By taking the inside-out approach, concussion patients can safely get back on their feet and back in the game faster.

Functional treatment means looking at the whole body

and all its complex, interconnected systems. In the same way, while all the treatments I discuss are valuable on their own, they work best when we bring them all together. I want you to say, as so many of my patients do, "Finally, something that works."

It's All About Your Gut!

The gut—meaning your small intestine and colon (large intestine)—is the center of your health universe. It's the bull's-eye, unequivocally. What makes it so central? Your gut is where what you eat becomes what nourishes you, but your gut does much more than that. It's a hugely important part of your immune system, for example. About 70 percent of your immune system's defense cells are found here. That makes a lot of sense, because you want to intercept any dangerous pathogens you might eat as quickly as possible. But what that also means is that anything that affects your gut also affects your immunity, much more than you might think.

Your gut, especially your colon, is where most of the trillions of bacteria that live in and on you reside. We call the overall population of bacteria (and also viruses, fungi, and parasites) the microbiome. The average human has about 100 trillion (yes, trillion) microbes just in their gut. That's about ten times more bacteria than you have cells in your entire body. In fact, while you have around 23,000 genes, the combined bacteria in your gut have about 3.3 million genes. It all adds up to carrying around three to five pounds of bacteria in your intestines.

When your bacteria outnumber your cells ten to one, ask yourself, who's really in charge here? It's your inner ecosystem. Far more than you may realize, your microbiome controls you. And far more than you may realize, what you do affects them. Every choice you make about your lifestyle and your diet influences your gut bacteria. A change in diet can shift the balance markedly within just a day.

Your microbiome contains at least five hundred different types of bacteria, including the kind we usually think of as bad, such as *Escherichia coli* and salmonella, bacteria that can cause food poisoning. Most of the bacteria in your gut are crucial to your very existence, because they help break down your food to release the nutrients. Some help digest carbohydrates and break down fiber. For example, bacterial enzymes break down fiber in the colon into short-chain fatty acids (SCFA) such as butyrate, which provides energy to cells in the intestines. That helps them grow and make a stronger gut wall that's less likely to allow toxins through it into the body. Your bacteria also manufacture some important nutrients, such as vitamin B12 and vitamin K.

A healthy, well-balanced microbiome contains some bad bacteria, but they're in the minority. They're held in check by all the neutral and good bacteria. They're there, but they can't usually get the upper hand and make you sick. It's another story when the microbiome isn't balanced—I'll talk about that later in this chapter.

Your gut is also sometimes called your second brain. That's because it has its own nervous system, called the enteric nervous system, and it produces a lot of the same neurotransmitter chemicals that your brain does. In fact, about 90 percent of the serotonin in your body is made in your gut, not your brain. We know that serotonin and other neurotransmitters influence mood, especially depression—many antidepressant drugs work by targeting serotonin in the brain. When your gut is dysfunctional, your brain may be as well. And the rest of your body may be affected too, because gut dysfunction causes inflammation—and if inflammation isn't controlled, it becomes chronic. And chronic inflammation is the underlying cause of a wide range of health problems, including asthma, atherosclerosis, type 2 diabetes, arthritis, liver problems, neurodegenerative diseases, and more.

You're never alone in life because you
always have your bacteria to talk to.

ARE YOUR GUTS LEAKY?

Your small intestine is around thirty feet long; if you opened it up and spread it out, it would cover a tennis court. So what makes it small? It's only about an inch in diameter and has about the thickness of a paper towel. The interior of the small intestine is tightly wrinkled into many, many circular folds. Each fold has thousands of finger-like projections called villi; one square inch of small intestine contains around 20,000 villi. Each villi has thousands of microvilli. The folds, villi, and microvilli vastly increase the total surface area of the small intestine so that you can absorb nutrients more efficiently. Think of the villi as shag carpeting (in fact, villi means "shaggy hair"). Just as shag carpeting grabs all the dirt that gets tracked onto it, the villi absorb nutrients from the digestive process and allow them to enter your bloodstream. The villi are coated with a mucosal membrane that keeps unwanted molecules from being absorbed.

Ordinarily, the folds, villi, and microvilli only absorb molecules of digested nutrients. They're held together very tightly at their junctions, which are open just enough to let nutrient molecules through. When the small intestine is stressed or damaged, however, the junctions can expand and open too wide. Think of it as taking out the grout between the tiles on your bathroom floor—water leaks through and damages the subflooring. Similarly, when the tight junctions in your intestinal wall loosen up, that lets larger molecules that haven't been completely broken down pass through and enter the bloodstream. Now you have gut hyperpermeability, better known as leaky gut syndrome.

What can make your gut stop protecting you? Lots of things. The top culprit is the Standard American Diet, which is based largely on processed foods that are high in calories, low in nutrition, and full of sugar, salt, bad fats, additives, and chemicals. The average American gets nearly half their calories from this sort of low-quality food every day. Your gut doesn't like that. Other possible causes of leaky gut include the following:

- Food allergies, gluten, and lactose
- Alcohol
- Overuse of nonsteroidal anti-inflammatory drugs (NSAIDs) such as aspirin and ibuprofen
- Antibiotics and other drugs, which kill off good bacteria
- Environmental toxins
- Pathogens such as *E. coli*
- Stress

Your body sees these large molecules as invaders and responds by activating your immune system, just like it would for a dangerous germ or toxin. The immune system goes on the attack. The immune response causes inflammation, which can in turn give you any of these symptoms:

- Digestive disorders such as gas, bloating, irritable bowel syndrome, and compromised liver function
- Joint pain, arthritis, and fibromyalgia
- Chronic fatigue syndrome
- Autoimmune diseases
- Skin problems such as eczema and hives
- Cognitive malfunction or "brain fog"

In addition, when your gut is compromised, your body is exposed to toxins that leak out. Toxins get broken down in the liver. Extra toxins mean a strain on the detoxification processes of the liver. They may not work as efficiently, meaning that toxins are hanging around in your body for longer than they should, causing inflammation.

In standard medicine, your doctor would look only at a symptom such as joint pain and prescribe an anti-inflammatory drug that will temporarily relieve the pain, at the risk of serious side effects. That's looking at the problem from the outside in. In functional nutrition, we look upstream to see what the underlying cause of the joint pain might be. Chances are good that leaky gut syndrome has something to do with it. Fixing the problem from the inside out by improving your diet and rebalancing your microbiome could be very helpful.

Gut on fire means brain on fire.

DYSBIOSIS AND WEIGHT GAIN

Dysbiosis means an imbalance in your gut bacteria. That can lead to all sorts of problems, primarily leaky gut syndrome. It can also lead to obesity. When your gut isn't absorbing nutrients well because the bacteria is out of balance, you feel hungry all the time. The digestive enzymes some bacteria make for you aren't being produced efficiently, so your ability to digest your food completely is thrown off. You start having cravings for carbohydrates and fats. You eat more and gain weight, but you're not really giving your body what it needs, which is the right bacteria. When patients come to me for help with weight loss, one of the first things we do is repair their gut by restoring a better balance of beneficial bacteria. Probiotic supplements will only help, however, if they have a healthy diet to feed on in the gut.

I tell my patients not to count calories but to count chemicals. If they're eating the Standard American Diet I talked about earlier, they will never lose weight or fix their dysbiosis—you can't expect miracles from your gut bacteria.

Or can you? Some very interesting recent research suggests that changing your gut bacteria alone can help you lose weight. The results come out of work on fecal transplants, where people with severe illness from a takeover of their gut by bad bacteria are given transplants of fecal material from healthy people. The good bacteria from the transplant can overwhelm the bad bacteria and restore a healthy balance in an amazingly short time. Research with lab animals and on people suggests that if the fecal transplant comes from someone who's overweight, the person getting the transplant can become overweight as well, even if they continue with their normal diet. By the same token, it seems to work the other way—bacteria from a skinny person makes a fat person lose weight. Does this mean that obesity has, at least in part, a bacterial basis? We don't know for sure yet, but it's possible that it does. And that means someday it might be possible to swap those fat bacteria for skinny ones. Don't try this at home, though.

DR. ROB'S SIX-STEP PROGRAM FOR GUT HEALTH

Over the years I've been in practice, I've treated hundreds of patients for dysbiosis and leaky gut syndrome. My protocol for healing the gut has six steps.

1. *Remove* chemicals (artificial sweeteners, additives, etc.), allergens, processed foods, soy, gluten, lactose, and sugar. Also remove bad bacteria through supplements containing concentrated aromatic oils (rosemary, thyme, sage, lemon balm, oregano, and natural antibacterial supplements such as berberine HCL). The Chinese herbs ginger, licorice, and skullcap are also helpful for removing bad bacteria.

2. *Replace* what was removed with an improved diet and lifestyle. Also replace missing digestive enzymes such as lipase, amylase, and protease; raise low stomach acid with supplements such as betaine HCL and pepsin.

3. *Reinoculate* the gut with probiotics to restore a better balance of good bacteria. (I'll explain more about probiotics later in this chapter.) A better balance can help relieve minor abdominal pain and discomfort.

4. *Regenerate and repair* the damage to the intestinal lining with supplements, including natural anti-inflammatories such as curcumin and omega-3 fatty acids. The amino acid glutamine is the primary energy source for the cells lining your intestines; taking supplements may really accelerate healing. Now's the time to add in B vitamins, vitamin D, selenium, and zinc. In serious cases, I recommend medical foods that can be used as

meal replacements. A medical food has balanced macronutrients (protein, carbohydrates, fats) in a formula with selected micronutrients (vitamins, minerals) and added ingredients such as the natural anti-inflammatory curcumin. I recommend products that contain selective kinase response modulators (SKRMs), which are helpful for restoring normal metabolic function. I also recommend supplements made with xanthohumol, a SKRM derived from hops. Xanthohumol blocks the expression of a protein called NF-kappa B, which plays an important role in preventing inflammation. It also provides potent antioxidant protection. At this stage, many of my patients also benefit from taking capsules containing specialized pro-resolving mediators (SPMs). These are derived from fish oil and are fantastically helpful for modulating inflammation naturally, without the side effects of anti-inflammatory drugs. (I'll discuss them in more detail later in this chapter. And I'll talk a lot more about inflammation in Chapter 4.)

5. *Retest* to see the gains that have been made and if any areas need further attention. Throughout the protocol, we test, assess, adjust, and reassess until we find what works for the patient. Supplements that help most people may not work as well in others. Everyone is different, and we use the tests to individualize the protocol. In functional nutrition,

we don't move on until we hit our goals.

6. *Retain* the gains with ongoing careful attention to diet, lifestyle, supplements, and the microbiome. I feel everyone should be taking a daily multivitamin with phytonutrients, along with two to four grams of a high-quality fish oil. Daily vitamin D supplements containing 2,000 to 5,000 IUs are also important. Ideally, you would have nine to thirteen daily servings of fruits and vegetables. Realistically, that's unlikely to happen on a sustainable basis. Instead, eat as many servings as you can each day and make up the difference with a high-quality organic green powder.

Another way to look at the six-step protocol is that it's Dr. Rob's Thirty-Day Gut Plan. Stick with it for a month, and chances are good that your gut will be in much better shape at the end.

Probiotics: Healing from the Inside

Probiotics are live microorganisms (bacteria) that confer a health benefit on the host when administered in adequate amounts. In other words, probiotics are beneficial bacteria in supplement form. By taking probiotic supplements, you can help restore a healthy balance of beneficial bacteria in your gut.

No shelf at the health food store is more confusing than

the probiotics display. The number of different products and what they contain can be very bewildering. It's also important to remember that the FDA doesn't regulate these products, so it's up to you to choose safe and effective ones.

Here's what to look for when you purchase a probiotic:

- Genus, species, and strain. Your gut contains hundreds of different kinds (genus and species) of bacteria. Not all are beneficial and most can't really be used in probiotics. That leaves just a handful of species that are truly capable of reaching and colonizing your gut when taken as probiotic supplement. The most common are bacteria in the family (genus) Lactobacillus and Bifidobacterium. Some strains of bacteria within these families are known to be particularly helpful (see the sidebar). Think of it this way: All dogs belong to the same species (Canis), but there's a big difference between a toy poodle and a pit bull. Same species, different strain.

- Minimum number of viable bacteria at the end of the shelf life. This is measured in colony forming units (CFU). The product should contain at least 10 billion CFU. All probiotic supplements start out with literally billions of live bacteria in them. As the product sits around, some of the bacteria naturally die off. That's normal, but you don't want to buy a dead product. Look for a product that reveals the expiration date, and don't buy a product that is near or past that date.

- The probiotic should come from a company that uses good manufacturing practices (GMP) to ensure quality, consistency, and safety. Look for a statement to that effect on the product label.

For normal maintenance of a good bacterial balance, I usually suggest taking one to two capsules a day. You should notice a difference in about thirty days.

Prebiotics

Probiotic supplements work best for rebalancing your bacteria if you give them a head start by also taking prebiotics. These are actually various types of nondigestible plant fiber that pass through the small intestine. When they arrive at the large intestine, they form a substrate that helps feed the beneficial bacteria and encourages them to recolonize the large intestine—sort of like fertilizer for the bacteria. They probably work by increasing your production of short-chain fatty acids (SCFA), which provide energy to the cells lining the colon. I suggest taking prebiotic supplements along with your probiotic supplements. Natural food sources of prebiotics include the skin of apples, bananas, beans, onions, garlic, Jerusalem artichoke, and chicory root. There's really no way you can eat enough of these foods to make a difference—supplements are the best approach.

SPMs

When you have dysbiosis or leaky gut syndrome, you also have inflammation. Your immune system is responding to what it sees as invaders, just as it would if you cut your finger or were sick with a virus. Your body is quick to start the inflammatory process, but slow to end it, especially if it's been going on for a long time. Recent breakthrough research on how inflammation gets resolved by the immune system has given us a powerful new tool: specialized pro-resolving mediators, or SPMs.

Specialized pro-resolving mediators, or SPMs, are a portion of the omega-3 fatty acid spectrum that have been shown to have a powerful effect on reducing inflammation. I'll explain how they work in detail in Chapter 4 on inflammation. For now, let's just say that when you take SPM supplements, your immune system is triggered to produce the natural chemical signals that stop the active inflammatory process and move your immune system toward the resolution process. The beauty of SPMs is that they work really well to reduce inflammation—as well as much more powerful (and dangerous) drugs—but with no side effects and no drug interactions. For speeding the repair and restoration of gut function that has been compromised by inflammation, SPMs are my go-to supplement.

LISTEN TO YOUR GUT

We often talk about our guts. We ask whether someone has the guts to do something. We do gut checks when making decisions. We have butterflies in our stomach or a bad feeling in our gut when we're nervous. We know intuitively that our guts affect everything else in our lives, including our emotions, and vice versa. Doesn't that mean you should be taking good care of your gut?

CASE STUDY: BACK ON THE JOB

・・・・・・

Undiagnosed or misdiagnosed gut problems have consequences beyond poor health. My patient Gail is a sad example. In her late teens, Gail had Lyme disease and needed heavy doses of antibiotics to get over it. The antibiotics seriously disrupted her microbiome, although this was never diagnosed or treated. She ended up taking a lot of ibuprofen to try to treat the aches and pains this caused, especially during her menstrual period. At the same time, Gail was sensitive to gluten, but this too was never diagnosed. The combination of all these factors finally gave her leaky gut syndrome. Now in her early thirties, for the past six years Gail had needed the bathroom so often and so unpredictably that she couldn't hold down a job. Her doctor accused her of abusing laxatives as part of an eating disorder. Her marriage failed. She came to me for functional nutritional counseling because she was so underweight. I could see right away that Gail's gut was clearly the issue. She needed an inside-out approach to restore it. We began by using berberine and other natural remedies to clear out the bad bacteria in her gut; we used probiotics and prebiotics to replace the bad bacteria with friendly ones. I put Gail on an elimination diet to take away gluten, dairy, soy, and other inflammatory foods and replace them with better choices for her. Gail responded with surprising speed. Within a couple of weeks, she had gained a few pounds, was sleeping better, and needed the bathroom less often. At the end of three months, she was getting close to her normal weight and looked and felt a lot better. The dark circles under her eyes were gone, and her hair and skin looked good. She told me she felt ready to go find a new job—and she did, just a few weeks later.

Your Knee Bone's Connected to...

Most of my patients first come to me to treat back pain, because chiropractic treatment has been shown to be very effective for this. The standard medical treatment for back pain is a good example of backward thinking. Most medical doctors simply prescribe rest and painkillers. To me, that's a Band-Aid on a bullet wound. Simply treating the pain won't solve the underlying cause of the problem. That shortsightedness is why so many people have chronic disease and chronic pain. In chiropractic, we treat the site of the pain in any musculoskeletal problem, but we know that is looking only at the symptom, not the system. More needs to be done to help the patient heal faster and completely, and more importantly, to help prevent future problems.

I use manual therapy ("adjustment") rehabilitation and a multitude of other chiropractic techniques to treat the painful area, but that's just the start. When the back or any other joint or muscle is chronically painful, the functional approach is to look at the whole system and start from the inside out. That means looking at two other areas: nutrition and movement. I use functional nutrition pathways to help repair the body. I also work with my patients to help them move better and have better awareness of their bodies (proprioception). If they're not moving well, they're ergonomically unsound, and they will have future problems. That's such an important aspect of overall health that I'll be discussing it in detail in Chapter 6.

The first step in treating a patient with back pain is to thoroughly assess the injury. The next step is to treat her pain and help her feel better. But long-term, I want to fix the structures, get patients healthy, bring their inflammation down, and make them move better. What I mean by that is our hips should be mobile. Our lower back should be very stable and not move too much. Most of my new patients have very tight hips and a lot of movement in the lower back.

The shoulders should also be mobile. I see a lot of patients who can't get their arms above their heads. It's only a matter of time before they have neck or mid-back injuries. It doesn't really matter what part of the body is painful or too mobile or not mobile enough. I'm going to take the functional approach and figure out what structure is injured and also what system is inflamed.

THE ARTHRITIS LINK

More than 52 million Americans suffer from arthritis, or to be more accurate, osteoarthritis. This is the kind of arthritis that doctors say comes from wear and tear. It doesn't. They're drastically wrong. Arthritis is in great part driven by a low-grade inflammatory process. We're learning that an autoimmune response to injury is what plays a key role in the onset of osteoarthritis.

A study at Stanford University found that low-grade inflammation isn't merely a symptom of osteoarthritic cartilage destruction—it's the trigger that causes it. The fraying of collagen (the main component of connective tissue) and the fraying of cartilage (the very strong, smooth material that cushions bones at joints) starts the inflammatory process. Many studies have shown that targeting the autoimmune response that occurs in the early development of osteoarthritis could keep the process from going any further.

If a joint becomes painful or is injured, and you don't do anything about it, it will probably become arthritic in another ten to fifteen years. The older you are and the more inflamed you are, the sooner arthritis will hit the joint.

When the cartilage in a joint is damaged, the body naturally responds with inflammation as a way to heal the injury. Unfortunately, the inflammatory process eats away at the collagen. The cartilage at the ends of the bones stops being very, very smooth and slippery and starts getting roughened and uneven. As the inflammation continues, often over the course of years, the cartilage deteriorates; it becomes rougher and more jagged. The joint becomes painful and swollen, and range of motion is limited—now you have osteoarthritis.

Arthritis starts with soft-tissue injuries. Your soft tissue is basically any part of the body that's not bone: muscles, tendons, ligaments, cartilage, and fascia. Tendons are the tough tissue that attach bones to muscles; ligaments are the tough fibers that hold joints together. Cartilage is the very smooth tissue found where bones come together in joints. And fascia are the thin sheaths of fibrous tissue that wrap around muscles and organs. Fascia hold your body together. I call fascia the Saran wrap of the body. If you've ever sliced a salmon, you've seen the white film between the muscles. Your fascia provide tensegrity—they hold the parts of your body together in a balance of tension and compression. The fascial system is the largest system in the body. In fact, it's the only system that touches every other system.

The extracellular matrix is the network that binds us together. It's made up of the fluid that fills the space between the cells of your body. Your cells "talk" to each other by sending biochemical messengers through the matrix. So, if you bang your knee, the joint sends out signals to the body saying the area has been injured and needs inflammatory cells to rush in and deal with the problem. That's perfectly normal and desirable—up to a point. The inflammation causes redness, swelling, warmth, and pain as your immune system clears away damaged cells and any invaders that might have gotten in. After the initial inflammatory response, the matrix should start to signal to the immune system that it's time to modulate the response. The swelling, redness, and warmth go down, and your knee hurts less. That's because the signal has told the immune system to stop sending white blood cells to the area and to start producing chemicals that will remodel the tissue and return you to normal.

One way the extracellular matrix does this is by producing enzymes called matrix metalloproteinases (MMP). They're your body's way of reducing inflammation by basically digesting the proteins created by the inflammatory process. Ordinarily, this is a good thing. However, overactivated release of MMPs can damage healthy tendons and cartilage. They end up digesting healthy collagen and connective tissue in the area. The injury itself can lead to overrelease, but the situation is made worse by poor diet and lifestyle.

The key to keeping an injury from getting worse is to

modulate the expression of MMPs. Otherwise, tendinitis (inflammation in a tendon) degenerates into tendinosis (chronic inflammation of the tendon). Research shows that overexpression of MMPs is the number-one reason why surgery for a torn rotator cuff fails. When we treat a soft tissue or connective tissue injury, we need to do everything we can to support healthy remodeling.

When you have a healthy extracellular matrix, you have healthy connective tissue. Your tendons, ligaments, fascia, and cartilage do what they're supposed to do without pain or inflammation. An unhealthy extracellular matrix leads to torn, weak, or relaxed tendons; soft-tissue injury; repetitive injury; and structural imbalances.

ACUTE INJURY

The first seventy-two hours of a soft-tissue injury are the acute phase. That's when you get swelling, redness, pain, spasms, and loss of function. Starting from day four all the way through to week eight, the injury is then in phase two, the healing phase. You still have some joint and muscle pain, and there's still some inflammation. Your range of motion may be compromised. What's important is that, by day four, tissue repair and remodeling has begun. That's when your body most needs to have proper treatment and good nutrition. Without that, the damaged joint is going to heal less than optimally. You'll have scar tissues and adhesions that will eventually lead to arthritis.

I see patients all the time who hurt a joint and don't come to see me until three or four weeks after the injury. They wait to see if the pain and loss of function will just somehow go away on their own, not realizing that they won't until it's too late. I always ask my patients, "Go away where? North, south, east, west? Where is it going?" The earlier musculoskeletal injuries are treated, the sooner healing can begin. An untreated injury can easily slide from being acute to being subacute to being chronic.

After about eight weeks, the injury is in phase 3, which is the wellness and prevention phase. By now you have, I hope, achieved optimum tissue remodeling and are back to normal in terms of pain and function. The goal at this point is to reduce the risk of reinjury and degeneration by continuing with good foundational nutrition.

Early Treatment

In the first seventy-two hours of an acute injury, nutrition matters. Patients need support that goes beyond what they can get even from a good diet. I recommend proteolytic enzyme supplements to my patients during this phase. Proteolytic enzymes such as trypsin, chymotrypsin, and bromelain are the enzymes the body naturally produces to digest proteins. I routinely use these enzymes to help patients with digestive problems (check back to Chapter 1 for more on this), but they have an additional use in treating injury. When they're taken on an empty stomach, these enzymes work systemically—that is, they work throughout the body to reduce inflammation. In particular, proteolytic enzymes break down the proteins in the blood that cause inflammation. They also remove fibrin, your body's natural clotting chemical, and bring down swelling. Essentially, proteolytic enzymes vacuum away a lot of the debris caused by the inflammatory response to an injury.

A number of other nutrients are safe, effective ways to address pain and inflammation. I like to use curcumin, the active ingredient in the spice turmeric (curry powder gets its yellow color from turmeric). Curcumin is a powerful anti-inflammatory compound that's particularly helpful for osteoarthritis. It works by blocking inflammatory pathways in much the same way as aspirin, but without the potentially dangerous side effects aspirin can cause. Other great natural anti-inflammatory supplements include Boswellia and ginger. They reduce inflammation, stimulate tissue repair, and regenerate damaged muscles. What I especially like about these supplements is that they work as well as NSAIDs such as aspirin and ibuprofen, but without the side effects of gastric upset and bleeding. They turn down the volume on pain and inflammation but don't shut them off. That's important, because early on in an injury, the inflammatory response is normal—you want it to occur as a natural step in the healing process.

Muscle injuries respond really well to supplemental calcium and magnesium. The typical multivitamin/mineral supplement has calcium and magnesium in a 2:1 ratio. If you're having muscle spasms, I recommend inverting the ratio and getting calcium and magnesium in a 1:2 ratio. Ordinarily, calcium helps muscles contract, while magnesium helps muscles relax. When you've got muscle soreness or spasms, you want the muscles to relax more than contract, so more magnesium is helpful. Magnesium also helps remove byproducts of exercise metabolism, such as lactic acid, that cause sore muscles. That's why Epsom salt soaks help with muscle soreness: Epsom salts are high in magnesium.

Phase 2 Treatment

In phase 2 of healing, the injury is now subacute—it's getting better and the tissues are remodeling. There's still some pain and inflammation, and range of motion is still compromised. This phase starts on day four and can last for weeks. Most tendon injuries, for instance, take four to six weeks to heal. What we want to do during this time is provide supplemental nutrients that will help prevent scar tissue formation, aid in healing, reduce the risk of reinjury, and control pain and inflammation. That means continuing with the same anti-inflammatory supplements as in the acute phase, but at gradually lower doses. At the same time, manual/chiropractic treatment, laser therapy (I'll talk more about that in Chapter 8), and therapeutic exercise help to restore range of motion and reduce pain.

IMPROVING MOVEMENT

· · · · · ·

An important concept in inside-out health is flexion movement versus flexion moment. Flexion moment means that you move with a hip hinge and hold your core tight. There's no movement at your lumbar (lower) spine. Flexion movement flexes the lumbar spine, which strains the layers of collagen that make up the spinal discs, the rubbery cushions between the individual vertebrae in your spine. When you have a lot of flexion movement, you release MMPs that damage the cartilage in the discs and cause inflammation, which in turn causes lower back pain. Eventually, this leads to a disc herniation: the disc material gets squished out of position and presses on the spinal nerves, causing intense pain. The problem is that flexion movement can go on causing lower back pain for a long time without showing up on an MRI. The discs look normal, with no bulges or displacements. Eventually, however, at least one disc will just give out, often without any external reason like lifting something heavy or being in a car accident. The reason is the long-term impact of inflammation from poor movement. Movement and exercise are so important for your health that I'll spend all of Chapter 6 discussing them.

Repairing the Damage

For phase 2 treatment, I like to use nutritional protocols that impact the MMPs. One supplement that's very effective as an anti-inflammatory is berberine. Another is a selective kinase response modulator (SKRMs). As I explained in Chapter 1, SKRMs are essentially enzymes that modulate the cellular signals that trigger inflammation.

Once the degeneration and inflammation have been stopped, the next step is to repair the injury. Think of it this way: When your house is on fire, you call the firemen and they put it out. The next day you don't call back the firemen; you call the general contractor. At this stage, you want to be rebuilding the injured area.

To rebuild tissue, you need to rebuild collagen. Collagen is a protein, and the building blocks of protein are amino acids. Supplements that contain specific amino acids, such as glycine, proline, taurine, and lysine, are effective. So is vitamin C, which is crucial to building collagen. To support connective tissue and joint stability, we want to add glucosamine, chondroitin, and MSM. These help build the shock-absorbing components of cartilage. These three supplements have been extensively studied and have been shown to be effective for knee and hip arthritis and for helping with spinal disc healing.

Another supplement that can be helpful is undenatured collagen type 2 (UC-II). This supplement is derived from chicken breastbones—it's the same collagen that's found in chicken soup. We used to think it was the antioxidants from the vegetables in chicken soup that made you feel better, but it's actually the collagen. Oral supplements of UC-II regulate the immune system and make it stop attacking the proteins that are normally found in healthy joints. Because it's undenatured—not changed in form—collagen from the chicken sternum goes right to the joint and gets absorbed, stopping the inflammatory signal there. It's very valuable for keeping an injured joint from becoming arthritic years down the line. In studies, UC-II increased the ability of people with knee arthritis to exercise longer and harder. When compared to glucosamine on several standard measurement scales, UC-II improved physical function and activities of daily living more. On the Lequesne Index for knee arthritis, for example, UC-II beat glucosamine by a factor of three.

We also want to use nutrients that modulate the production of matrix metalloproteinases. A compound called THIAA (tetrahydro iso-alpha acids), derived from hops, is a very valuable supplement for inhibiting MMP inflammation. It works by modulating kinase activity and shifting it toward good joint health. Among its many advantages is the lack of side effects and interactions. Overall, THIAA reduces swelling in acute inflammation and inhibits bone and cartilage degradation in chronic inflammation.

A product from Metagenics called OsteoVantiv® combines a clinically effective dose of UC-II with a proprietary form of THIAA. The combination has very powerful anti-inflammatory effects. It's been shown to decrease injury and swelling in both acute and chronic conditions.

MMPs actually come in several different types. THIAA works on all of them. Berberine, selenium, and folic acid work individually on different MMP types. When these supplements are taken together, they work synergistically to modulate MMPs. Berberine, taken with THIAA, works synergistically to modulate one type of MMP. Selenium and folic acid help modulate other types. Adding in zinc and biotin helps reduce inflammation from other chemical messengers.

Phase 3: Optimal Healing and Avoiding Reinjury

In phase 3 of healing, the pain, inflammation, and limited motion are gone. Now you want to achieve optimum tissue remodeling and avoid reinjury. This is best done by maintaining good foundational nutrition. At this point, I recommend my Super 5 nutrients:

- Multivitamin/mineral complex with additional phytonutrients—one tablet daily
- Omega-3 fatty acids (fish oil)—2 grams daily
- Vitamin D—2,000 IU daily
- Probiotics—two capsules daily
- Phytonutrient green drink—once daily

Vitamin D is particularly important. Just about everyone is deficient in vitamin D because we get very little natural sunlight on the skin, which is crucial for manufacturing vitamin D in the body. That leads to a lot of health problems. We've found that virtually everybody who has a susceptibility to musculoskeletal injuries is also deficient in vitamin D. Adding at least 2,000 IU daily can help with healing and may help prevent another injury down the line.

A lot of manufacturers offer green drink powders. The quality varies a lot from brand to brand. To avoid wasting time and money, I recommend using Nutri-Dyn Dynamic Fruits and Greens.

JOINT OR MUSCLE?

When my patients ask me if their problem is from a joint or a muscle, I always answer, "Yes." One of the most important things we've come to understand is that we mean it when we say the musculoskeletal *system*. The functional medicine approach is to look at systems, and no system is more interconnected than your bones and your muscles. If you have back pain or a problem with repeated ankle injuries, you're dealing with both muscles and bones. The problems don't exist in isolation from each other. Let's say you have a torn ligament. Ligaments connect bone to bone within a joint. Because you have a ligament injury, the joint is now a bit unstable and you're more likely to get a bone injury down the line.

Take a sprained ankle, for instance. The most common ankle injury—in fact, it's the most common sports injury— is a sprain to the anterior talofibular ligament. If that happens to you, you've opened a Pandora's box of problems. This sort of sprain has an 80 percent recurrence rate.

When you sprain your ankle, you walk with a limp for weeks. Even after the ankle has healed and you've gone back to normal, you really haven't healed completely. Your brain has been retrained to think that the abnormal way you walked with the sprained ankle is now the normal way to walk. When that happens, your body is thrown off balance. The gluteus maximus (the muscle you sit on) on that side gets shut off. That weakens your hip on that side. Your quadriceps (the large muscle in the front of your thigh) tighten up. You're now more susceptible to spraining the ankle again or having a knee injury.

That whole cascade of problems could be avoided with better treatment that sees the ankle as part of the whole musculoskeletal system right from the start. The conventional treatment for a sprained ankle is to ice it and rest it. While icing helps reduce the swelling a bit right after the injury, it's not really helpful after that. And resting the joint is exactly the wrong approach. What's needed is proprioceptive treatment to restore normal motion. If you immobilize the joint, you reach a point where you can't even put your foot down. How does immobilizing the joint help get the blood flowing through it? You need that to flush out the byproducts of inflammation and carry them away from the injured area. Instead, you should be getting quality modalities of adjustment immediately. In chiropractic, we use soft-tissue adjustment, lasers, and rehab exercises.

The standard medical treatment for the inflammation of a musculoskeletal injury is anti-inflammatory drugs like aspirin and ibuprofen. I've already talked about the risk of these drugs and the many more effective natural supplements that are good alternatives, like proteolytic enzymes. With functional treatment, we can cut the time for healing an ankle sprain in half. We can also reduce the risk of recurrence from 80 percent to 20 percent.

Building Musculoskeletal Health

In functional nutrition, we see that the bones and joints are connected to everything else. If the framework isn't healthy and strong, neither is anything else. Therapeutic lifestyle changes that incorporate the right amount of movement are great for proactively building your musculoskeletal health. Therapeutic lifestyle changes mean stress reduction, better diet, more exercise, and the right supplements. You don't have to become a gym rat; you just have to move more. Today, we realize that sitting for hours in front of the computer or the TV has a lot of bad impacts. In fact, we now say sitting is the new smoking. Every hour you sit is equivalent to smoking a cigarette. Stop sitting and move more. I like to encourage my patients to aim for ten thousand steps a day. I also encourage my patients to look at things like their computer work areas. I see a lot of injuries from bad ergonomics—things arranged inefficiently or awkwardly make you put your body into unnatural positions that can cause problems like carpal tunnel syndrome or neck stiffness.

Your bones are the framework for the rest of your body. They need to be as strong as possible to support everything else. Your bones are made mostly of calcium, so you need plenty of it, but good bone health depends on more than calcium.

For supplementing, the best form of calcium by far is microcrystalline hydroxyapatite concentrate, shortened to MCHC. It's made from pure bovine bone. MCHC has organic constituents to give it the highest level of absorbability. Supplements made with calcium carbonate or calcium citrates aren't good choices—they're simply not absorbed very well. In addition to MCHC, supplements of vitamin D, boron, and magnesium improve absorbability.

Your bones are dynamic and alive—they're not like the dry bones of the skeleton you remember from biology class. Your bones are constantly changing and being remodeled. In the bone matrix, cells called osteoblasts lay new bone down; other cells called osteoclasts break down old and damaged bone in a process called resorption. As both men and women age, the osteoclasts start to outnumber the osteoblasts and bone density goes down. At any given time, your skeleton has between one and two *million* remodeling sites—your bones are in constant activity. At age forty, most women start to lose about 1 percent of their bone density a year. Men start to lose about 2 percent of their bone density at that age, but they start with much heavier, thicker bones to begin with, so the lifetime loss of their bone density usually isn't very noticeable and doesn't cause problems. That's not to say men can't get osteoporosis—they can and they do. That's why building bone strength earlier in life and maintaining it throughout your lifetime is important for everyone.

When women reach menopause, the drop in their estrogen production can allow the osteoclasts to really get the upper hand, leading to rapid loss of bone density. Over time, this can lead to osteoporosis—thin, brittle bones that break easily. Osteoporosis can be very painful and crippling. The best way to avoid it is to have strong bones to begin with.

The bones you build in adolescence and early adulthood are the bones that have to carry you the rest of your life. They need to be as strong and dense as possible, because after age thirty there's no more building, and after forty there's only slow bone loss. That's why I recommend calcium supplements for all women, starting in adolescence. This is particularly important for young female athletes. On the one hand, exercise builds bone at that age. On the other hand, many girls and young women suffer from female athlete triad (FAT). They train too hard and often diet too much (especially in weight-conscious sports like dance and gymnastics), to the point where they develop three distinct but related conditions: disordered eating (a range of poor nutritional behaviors), amenorrhea (irregular or absent menstrual periods), and osteoporosis. Parents, trainers, and teammates need to be alert for FAT before the athlete does serious long-term damage to her health. All young women, not just athletes, should be taking calcium supplements to make sure they build up their bones as much as possible.

Bone strength depends on more than just calcium. Vitamin D and vitamin K play an important part; so does a good diet with adequate amounts of protein. Even when all that's in place, however, menopausal women still face accelerated bone loss. If there's a family history of osteoporosis, the bone loss is likely to be even faster. Older women can improve their bone density somewhat with bone remodeling supplements. One formulation I like is called Ostera, made by Metagenics. It contains vitamin K, vitamin D, berberine, and a SKRM. When taken with a high-quality calcium supplement, it can help slow bone loss.

In addition to supplements, calcium should also come from the diet. Dairy products are high in calcium, but you don't need to drink milk to obtain more calcium in your diet. In fact, I recommend against it, because the calcium in milk isn't that absorbable. A better approach is to eat lots of leafy green vegetables and nuts, which are also high in calcium. Research shows that a Mediterranean-style food plan is a good approach to getting the calcium, protein, fat, and other nutrients that help keep bones healthy.

What's not in the Mediterranean diet? Sugar and processed foods. In the Mediterranean diet, you drink water and the occasional glass of wine. What you don't drink is soda—and that's an important reason for why the Mediterranean diet helps with bone health. The phosphoric acid found in both regular and diet soda can interfere with the mineralization process that builds up bone. Your body combines phosphorus with calcium to make bone. When you drink a lot of soda, the phosphoric acid gives you more phosphorus than your body needs. For reasons we don't fully understand yet, that can throw off the calcium/phosphorus balance and lead to excess bone loss. The problem is especially bad for cola addicts. A major study at Tufts University showed that women who drink three or more cola sodas a day have reduced bone density in the hip. Let me just remind you that older adults who break a hip usually end up in nursing homes for months on end—and many die there.

I like coffee. I don't have a problem with my patients drinking it, but there's a limit. Caffeine from any source—including colas—can interfere with calcium absorption. For bone health, keep the caffeine down to a max of four cups of coffee a day, and skip the colas.

Supplements and diet aren't always enough to slow bone loss and avoid osteoporosis. You also need to do weight-bearing exercises that puts a little stress on your bones. The stress stimulates the production of osteoblasts and helps lay down new bone. Yoga class is great, but it doesn't do much for your bone density. You need to put more weight on your bones. The best exercises for this tends to be high-impact, like dancing, hiking, jogging, playing tennis, and stair climbing. If you can't do high-impact exercise, go for low-impact weight-bearing exercise. The rower, elliptical, and stair-stepping machines are good choices. So are water aerobics.

In my view, the best exercise you can do for your bones is taking a brisk walk. You already know how to walk, you don't have to join a gym to do it, and it's free. With every step you take, you're lifting your body weight and also giving your cardiovascular system a workout.

Inflammation anywhere in the body ramps up osteoclast activity as well. For women at risk of osteoporosis, damping down chronic inflammation is really important—I'll discuss this in detail in Chapter 4.

CASE STUDY: ARTHRITIS IS NOT INEVITABLE

· · · · · ·

My patient Josie, a retired schoolteacher, came to me because she had painful arthritis in her left shoulder, spine, and both knees. She didn't think I could help her much After all, she said, her mother and grandmother had arthritis everywhere as well. Wasn't it inevitable that she would, too? I told her genetics did play a role in osteoarthritis, but it's a small one. Diet and lifestyle are much bigger factors, which means we can help arthritis from the inside out. Josie was only in her early sixties. She was definitely willing to do what it took to avoid a future of worsening pain and limited mobility. We started by doing lab tests for inflammatory markers in the blood. As I expected, they were high. Josie was overweight from a combination of a diet high in processed foods and not a lot of activity. We needed to tackle her arthritis from several different directions, because her diet and lifestyle were basically just adding fuel to the fire. The first step was to improve her diet and reduce her inflammation from that cause. She cut out wheat, corn, dairy foods, peanut butter, and fried foods and substituted foods that help with inflammation. I also had her start taking a good multivitamin with minerals, extra vitamin D, a daily green drink, and a daily dose of SPMs. Within a couple of weeks, she had lost weight and was feeling better in general—her mild depression had lifted and her pain was better. I got her to add in gentle exercise just by walking more. That seems counterintuitive for someone with arthritis in both knees, but our joints are meant to move. Not using them is actually abusing them. We also began standard chiropractic rehab protocols for arthritis. At the end of three months, Josie was feeling substantially better. She had lost twenty pounds without really dieting, and she found the activities of daily living easier. She is now looking ahead to an active future and enjoying her retirement.

Toxins, Toxins, Toxins

It's a toxic world out there, but most people don't realize it. Patients often come to me with symptoms like dark circles under the eyes, all sorts of digestion problems, muscle and joint pain, being overweight or underweight, weakness, depression, headaches, brain fog, and memory and concentration problems. But mostly they come to me for fatigue, the number-one complaint in all of health care.

When we first talk, most patients attribute their problems to a specific cause. They say they have rings under their eyes, for instance, because they're not getting enough sleep. Maybe, but probably not. When patients consistently have fairly general symptoms like fatigue or vague digestive problems, it's time to take the functional approach and look at what's going on in their systems. And often, what's going on is an overload of toxins.

Just about all of us carry around a hidden load of chemicals and toxins we've picked up from our environment. We breathe in car exhaust, paint fumes, and air pollution. We absorb mercury from seafood and, unfortunately, sometimes lead from our drinking water. We're exposed to toxins from plastics, fabric softeners, fire retardants, household cleaning products, and all the other chemicals we encounter as an ordinary part of modern life.

DR. ROBINS

You can't be a clean fish in a dirty bowl.

According to a 2004 study from the Centers for Disease Control, most people in America are routinely exposed to 212 different toxins. Of those, six were found most commonly in the blood and urine:

1. BPA (bisphenol A), used very extensively in packaging and plastics
2. PBDEs (polybrominated diphenyl ethers), flame retardant widely used in carpet, curtains, upholstery, and household furnishings such as cushions and pillows
3. PFCs (perfluorochemicals) and PFOA (perfluorooctanoic acid), used in nonstick cookware and also in outdoor clothing and food packaging, including

microwave popcorn bags and pizza boxes

4. Acrylamide, found in coffee and carbohydrates that have been cooked at a high temperature, such as potato chips and French fries

5. Mercury, found in some seafood and shellfish, especially swordfish, mackerel, and canned white tuna

6. MTBE (methyl tert-butyl ether), used as a gasoline additive and found in secondhand smoke.

Let's take a closer look at some of these.

BPA is everywhere. It's on credit card receipts, for instance. It's also in brochures, magazines, bus and train tickets, food wrappers, airplane boarding passes, even toilet paper and paper towels. It's used to line food cans, particularly those containing tomato sauce.

High levels of BPA in the body are linked to coronary artery disease, type 2 diabetes, and liver enzyme abnormalities. They're also linked to birth defects and an increased risk of miscarriage. BPA is also an ovarian toxin that blocks estrogen and may be the underlying cause of some cases of infertility and ovarian cancer. There's some evidence that BPA is also linked to low testosterone in men. People with high levels of BPA also have more body fat and a greater risk of obesity. BPA increases body fat by altering insulin sensitivity, slowing metabolism, causing inflammation, and decreasing levels of the hormone adiponectin, which regulates fat burning. Lowering BPA levels has been studied as a primary treatment for obesity. PBDEs can have an effect on the thyroid gland and the liver and may also affect neurobehavior and the immune system. PFCs are linked to cancer and birth defects. Acrylamide is linked to cancer in lab animals; the World Health Organization says acrylamide is a human health concern. Mercury is a powerful neurotoxin. MTBE may cause cancer. Fortunately, this additive hasn't been used in gasoline since 2006, so you're more likely to be exposed to it from secondhand smoke.

A number of widely used chemicals can have endocrine-disrupting effects, meaning they affect your hormones. These chemicals can imitate your own hormones, increase or decrease the production of some hormones, and interfere with hormone signaling. You don't want these substances in your body.

I've already talked about how BPA in plastics can block estrogen. Lots of other chemicals are endocrine disrupters, including dioxin, a dangerous, long-lived chemical that is used in thousands of industrial processes (and is also found in tampons); phthalates, a group of chemicals widely used in plastics of all sorts; and atrazine, a herbicide used on corn.

And then there are the toxins we don't know much about, singly or in combination. According to the FDA, the average person uses nine personal care products daily. In total, those nine products contain about 126 chemical ingredients. The time it takes for the chemicals in personal care products to enter the blood stream is twenty-six seconds. We don't really know what happens when the different ingredients, each considered reasonably safe, combine in your body.

TOXINS AND DETOXIFICATION

In addition to all their other possible effects, the accumulated toxins in your body reduce your energy level by damaging the mitochondria, the tiny power plants in your cells. In my view, accumulated toxins in the body are why so many of us feel tired all the time.

Clearly, carrying around a lot of toxins in your body isn't good for you. Lightening the toxin load makes a lot of sense—it's a great way to heal the body from the inside out.

Detoxification—getting rid of toxins—happens in two ways. First, decrease your exposure. OK, I appreciate that in today's world, that's not always easy. Still, without too much effort you can lower your exposure to a lot of the chemicals all around us. You can switch to safer personal care products and household cleaning products (check out the Environmental Working Group at ewg.org for good choices). You can eat organic foods to reduce your exposure to pesticides and eat fresh foods instead of canned to reduce your exposure to BPA. You can avoid secondhand smoke. You can replace your nonstick cookware and make popcorn in the air popper. Install a reverse-osmosis water filter for your drinking water.

Just reducing your exposure won't help you get rid of the toxins that have built up in your body. For that, you need to follow a detoxification program.

LIVER FUNCTION AND DETOXIFICATION

To understand why detoxing on a regular basis (spring and fall) is so important, we have to take a detour into your liver.

Your liver is the largest organ inside your body (your skin is your largest organ of all), weighing about three pounds (a bit more than your brain). It's where 75 percent of your detoxification takes place—the rest happens in your gut. Your liver not only removes wastes; it also regulates the amounts of glucose, fat, and protein that enter your blood stream. It produces the clotting factors you need to clot your blood properly. It's where cholesterol comes from. And the liver is where the nutrients absorbed by the intestines get converted into forms that can be used by the body. In all, your liver has over five hundred different functions!

Your liver gets rid of endotoxins: the waste products that naturally accumulate from your normal metabolism. For example, your liver is where the hemoglobin from old, worn-out red blood cells is processed and removed from your body. To put that in perspective, every second of every day, your body destroys 2.5 million red blood cells out of the 25 trillion or so you have. Your liver is kept busy just handling your day-to-day detoxification.

What happens when you add to the load by asking your liver to also remove exotoxins? These are toxins that aren't part of your normal metabolism, like alcohol, the breakdown products of pharmaceuticals, all the additives found in processed foods, and all the other toxins you absorb from your environment. Your liver copes as well as it can, but it's stressed. Normal detoxification takes longer, which means waste products hang around your body longer than they should. That's not good. When your liver is kept too busy detoxifying you, its other functions may not work as well as they should.

Removing waste products in your liver is a two-phase process. Phase 1 is called detoxification. It starts with a family of enzymes collectively called the cytochrome p450 system. Fat-soluble toxins—just about all toxins are fat-soluble—are carried into the liver through the bloodstream. In the liver, these enzymes react with the toxins through a variety of different pathways. They start breaking them down into less complex molecules that are water-soluble. In the process, damaging byproducts called free radicals are released. A healthy liver can squelch free radicals quickly, before they can do any real harm. An overloaded, sluggish liver can't.

The breakdown products of phase 1 then move to phase 2, also called conjugation. In this phase, six different pathways take the phase 1 products and attach (conjugate) them to water-soluble molecules that let them be carried out of the body in the urine or the feces.

The breakdown and conjugation phases need a lot of nutrients to function properly. During breakdown, for instance, you need almost all the B vitamins; during conjugation, you need plenty of amino acids.

In a healthy liver, phase 1 and phase 2 are synchronized. When the liver gets overloaded, or if you take in a lot of caffeine or alcohol, the two phases can get out of sync. Phase 1 can happen too quickly for phase 2 to handle. That means lots of extra free radicals are damaging your liver while toxins and partially detoxified molecules continue to circulate in your body. I'm a basketball guy, so I tend to think in basketball terms. When your detox phases are out of sync, it's like Lebron James is phase 1. He's throwing basketballs full of detoxified molecules at Rob Silverman, who is trying to catch them and get them onto the right pathways. The problem is, Lebron is throwing them too quickly, so Rob can't catch them. Some of the basketballs zoom right past me. They get back to Lebron eventually, but in the meantime they're bouncing around and knocking things over. Or maybe Lebron is just throwing at a normal pace, but Rob is having a bad day and can't catch everything. Either way, when the two phases aren't working well, your body suffers. An important part of doing a detox program is getting your detoxification and conjugation phases working at the right levels again.

DOING DETOX

Should you do a detox program? I highly recommend it, especially if you regularly have one or more of these common symptoms:

- Fatigue, lethargy, weakness
- Depression
- Headaches, irritability
- Cognitive problems such as brain fog or memory issues
- Difficulty concentrating
- Generalized muscle aches
- Dark circles under the eyes
- Digestion problems
- Elimination problems
- Muscle and joint pain
- Overweight or underweight
- Skin problems and rashes

Detoxing isn't a do-it-yourself project. To do it safely and well, you want to do it with professional help and follow a program that supports the body's detox systems with the right supplements.

Here's what happens when you detox. My big household responsibility is taking out the trash every night. Think of the liver as your garbage bag. Phase 1 is when all the garbage gets put in the bag. Phase 2 is when you take the bag out and put it in the garbage can for the sanitation engineers to take away. If I get lazy and forget to take out the garbage, what happens? It begins to rot and stink. That's your liver if you don't detox.

The Ten-Day Detox

I usually have my patients do a ten-day detox program following a modified elimination diet and also using a medical food powder to give them all the nutrients needed for phase 1 and phase 2. Because about 25 percent of your detoxification happens in your gut, I also have patients take a probiotic formula. The medical food I prefer is called UltraClear Renew, made by Metagenics. I've used it with over a thousand patients and achieved fabulous, long-lasting results. UltraClear contains all the nutrients we know you need to fuel the detoxification pathways in the liver. It also contains potassium citrate to keep the body at the proper pH and flush water-soluble toxins out.

A ten-day detox is a commitment to your health. To get the most from it, plan ahead a bit. If you usually consume a lot of caffeine or eat a lot of sugar, start cutting back at least a week before you plan to start your detox. If at all possible, don't schedule any business trips or big events during the ten days of your detox. Plan to take it easy during this time. You can still go to the gym, but avoid strenuous exercise.

The ten-day detox has three steps.

Step 1 is initial clearing. During the first four days, you'll gradually eliminate potentially allergenic foods such as soy and dairy products. You'll also gradually increase the amount of UltraClear you take in as a nutritional beverage. During the detox, you'll be avoiding caffeine, alcohol, and soda. Instead, you'll be drinking lots of pure water, pure apple and pear juice, and mild herbal teas. Your food choices during this step become more limited, but don't worry. A key point about the entire ten days is that you should never be hungry. You can eat all you want of the allowed foods. Most people lose some weight when they detox, but that's not the goal—it's just a side benefit. We're removing chemicals, not calories.

Step 2 is metabolic detoxification. For days five through seven, you'll eat a more restricted diet of high-quality protein such as fish and lentils, along with lots of apples, pears, salad, and green vegetables. You'll also be drinking the UltraClear nutritional beverage. These few days can be challenging, but almost all my patients get through them.

Step 3 is reintroduction. On days eight and nine, you slowly reintroduce foods such as rice, nuts, berries, and oatmeal. You also reduce the amount of the nutritional beverage. On day ten, you're done! Now you can start slowly adding back other foods. I recommend adding only one or two new foods a day and being alert to reactions during the next two days.

I ask my patients to check in with me every couple of

days while they're detoxing. Sometimes we need to tweak the program a bit to individualize it. Some patients find it hard to skip alcohol during the detox. In fact, one of my patients told me he'd rather die than not have his evening cocktail. I told him, "That might actually happen if you don't do the detox." He finally agreed and found that it really wasn't so hard. In fact, it made him realize that he didn't really need that cocktail every evening after all.

At the end of the detox, my patients look and feel better. The dark rings under their eyes go away, their hair looks better, their skin looks better, they have an increase in energy, and they lose a little weight. All those benefits occur from treating not the symptoms but the system.

DETOX OR CLEANSE?

. . . . . .

Cleansing programs have become very popular. Even though many cleansing diets label themselves with names like "Three-Day Super Cleanse," they don't help you detoxify. Most cleanses turn out to be water or juice fasts or programs that supposedly clean out the bowel. A cleanse to me is just one big poop. Cleanses such as juice fasting are high in sugar and low in calories, especially protein calories. What does that do? It speeds up phase 1 in the liver and slows down phase 2. Cleanses don't help the liver—in fact, by depriving you of the protein and nutrients your liver needs to function well, you're actually stressing it. A cleanse isn't a detox and a detox isn't a cleanse.

The hormone estrogen is broken down and cleared from the body in the liver. Making sure this pathway is working smoothly is extremely important for all women, because excess estrogen can trigger breast and other cancers. I already mentioned that BPA is an estrogen blocker, which means it keeps your natural estrogen from being used by your body; the excess ends up floating around and getting broken down in the liver. Other sources of exogenous estrogen include birth control pills and hormone replacement therapy.

The primary active form of estrogen in your body is estradiol. When estradiol is metabolized in your liver, it breaks down into estrone. Just to complicate things, estrone comes in three different forms. The good estrone form (2-hydroxy estrone) has a protective effect against breast cancer. The bad estrone form (16-hydroxy estrone) can damage breast tissue. And the really bad estrone (4-hydroxy estrone) can trigger breast cancer (and also prostate cancer in men). Some people are just genetically prone to making more of the bad estrones.

To help your body break down estrogen into the safest forms, first, avoid estrogen disrupters whenever possible. After that, eat a lot of cruciferous vegetables, such as cabbage, broccoli, and kale. Substances called indoles in these foods can tip estrogen detoxification toward the good estrone. Excess estrogen is excreted in the bowel.

A diet high in fiber will move things through the bowel quickly and keep excess estrogen from being reabsorbed. Here's another place where probiotics can be helpful. Some unfriendly bacteria in the gut produce an enzyme called beta glucuronidase. High levels of this enzyme disrupt your ability to detoxify natural and exogenous estrogen. To minimize the impact of the bacteria that produce beta glucuronidase, take a good probiotic supplement to increase the good bacteria in your gut and overwhelm the bad ones. Be sure to get a good supply of B vitamins from a daily supplement. B vitamins are needed to methylate estrogen breakdown products, which helps remove them efficiently.

Heavy Metal Detox

Heavy metals are substances such as lead, mercury, and cadmium, and they are very harmful to the body—among other things, they're neurotoxins. Lead can come from old paint, household dust, and water contaminated by lead pipes. Cadmium and mercury are industrial byproducts—they enter your body through air and water pollution. Cadmium is also found in tobacco smoke. Your body has a hard time getting rid of heavy metals. The natural mechanism is an enzyme called metallothionein, which carries heavy metals out of your cells and transports them to the liver, where they get detoxified and then excreted. The process isn't that efficient, however, mostly because having such high levels of heavy metals is something our bodies really aren't meant to cope with. To help the enzyme work as well as possible, I recommend phytonutrients derived from hops (humulus lupulus), pomegranates, prune skin extract, and watercress. In addition, you need good amounts of the calcium, magnesium, selenium, and zinc.

GETTING DOWN TO BASICS

Once your detoxification system is back on track, it's time to focus on the final piece of the puzzle: your pH. I like to think of this as phase 3 of detoxification. Your pH is a measure of your body's alkalinity or acidity. A pH of 7 is neutral; above 7 is alkaline, and below 7 is acidic. Your body likes to be slightly on the alkaline side, ideally between 7.0 and 7.4, and it will go to great lengths to keep you that way, including robbing calcium from your bones. I've found with my patients that those who have low pH tend to have more musculoskeletal disorders. One reason is that their bodies steal calcium from the bones and the extracellular matrix to neutralize the tendency toward acidity.

Among other benefits, when you're on the alkaline side, your body has an easier time eliminating toxins through the kidneys. A good diet with lots of green vegetables and plenty of pure water helps keep you alkaline. In addition, the supplement potassium citrate helps raise your pH a bit. This is a supplement that has a long history of safe use in hospitals. I usually suggest a minimum dose of 600 mg daily.

CASE STUDY: TEENAGERS OR TOXINS?

· · · · · ·

When Daphne, a forty-six-year-old single mom came to me, it was because she constantly had mysterious aches and pains all over her body. She was gaining weight, her energy was nonexistent, and her digestion was a mess. She put it all down to the stress of raising three teenaged girls by herself.

After we reviewed her medical history and nutritional status, I knew stress wasn't the problem. Toxins were. Daphne had grown up in a big city famed for its smog. She loved to garden, but it turned out she lived next to a major highway. She was breathing exhaust fumes all the time, especially when she was outdoors in the garden. Her accumulated toxin load was showing up not just in her aches and pains but in her thinning hair, headaches, inability to lose weight, and the dark circles under her eyes.

Daphne wanted me to give her chiropractic treatments for her aching body, but what we ended up doing was a twenty-eight-day detoxification, along with some therapeutic lifestyle changes. That takes commitment, but Daphne was ready to try anything to feel better. At the end of her detox, she felt almost reborn. She was ten pounds lighter, her headaches were gone, the dark circles had disappeared, and her skin and hair looked great. She told me that she was much calmer around her kids, and family tensions had really eased. Her next step is to find a new place to live, as far from toxins in the air as possible.

Inflammation Nation

*You can't buy health, but it's a great
savings account to have.*

Inflammation is your body's normal response to injury or attack. Let's say you cut your finger. Your immune system is immediately triggered to fight off any dangerous germs the cut lets in. Or let's say you sprained your ankle. Your immune system is immediately triggered to deal with the internal damage. White blood cells pour into the area to kill off germs and remove debris; chemical signals tell your body to activate other defenses, like making your blood clot faster.

In both cases—injury or attack—you then get the classic signs and symptoms of inflammation. The area becomes red, warm to the touch, painful, and swollen. In the case of your ankle, your range of motion is also restricted. After a while, your immune system has pretty much done its job, and the inflammation gradually goes away.

That's the normal response to inflammation, because it comes from normal daily life. But what happens when you're constantly exposed to attack just from the environment around you? From your diet? From having a chronic condition or infection? You're inflamed all the time—your body is on fire. It's just that because the inflammation is happening inside you, you don't see the most obvious signs. But inflammation is harming you from the inside out—and putting out the flames also has to happen from the inside out.

CHRONIC INFLAMMATION

Low-grade systemic inflammation, or chronic inflammation, is what I call meta-inflammation. Just about everyone now suffers from this, because we're constantly exposed to toxins, because so many of us eat a bad diet full of sugar and processed foods, because so many of us are overweight, and because so many of us have leaky gut syndrome and other pro-inflammatory conditions.

When you're constantly suffering from meta-inflammation, you're not actually fighting off a disease or repairing an injury. Instead, your body is constantly perpetuating the inflammation, rather than resolving it. That's because while your immune system can fight off a specific invader or repair an injury and then calm down again, when you're constantly being exposed to an inflammatory agent that won't go away, such as high levels of the hormone insulin in your bloodstream, your immune system never gets a rest.

The long-term damage of meta-inflammation leads to a lot of chronic disease. Meta-inflammation damages the linings of your arteries, for instance, and plays a big role in coronary artery disease and stroke. Inflammation also plays a huge role in arthritis, Alzheimer's disease, autoimmune diseases, fibromyalgia, and many other life-limiting chronic problems. The inflammatory signals your body is sending all the time also cause the membranes in your body's cells to become unstable.

Think of it this way: You need a fire to cook your food, but if you don't pay attention, that fire can get out of control and burn down the house.

DR. ROB-ISM

NSAIDs decrease pain but impair healing.
Nutraceuticals decrease pain and promote healing.

Inflammation is responsible for pain and tissue destruction in almost all my patients; it's associated with virtually every chronic disease. I often use the acronym STAMP when I talk about inflammation—after all, we want to STAMP it out. Here's what it stands for:

S is stress, sleep, and sugar.

T is toxins.

A is allergies, acidity, and autoimmune diseases.

M is microbes, mitochondria, and methylation.

P is processed food and poor posture.

Let's take these one at a time.

Stress, Sleep, and Sugar

With too much stress, too little sleep, and way too much sugar is the way most of us live today. We're all under a lot of stress as we juggle family and work. Chronic stress is great for causing chronic inflammation, because chronic stress raises the amount of cortisol you produce. Cortisol is the hormone your body makes when you're under stress. Among other things, it raises your blood sugar, increases the amount of fat in your blood, raises your blood pressure and makes your heart beat faster, revs up your nervous system, and heightens your immune response. That's fine when you're fighting off zombies, because you want that burst of energy stress can give you in a dangerous situation. But when you're chronically stressed and always have high cortisol levels, that contributes to meta-inflammation. Among other things, chronic stress lowers your immune function. That means any inflammation you might have from an illness or injury lingers on longer.

Chronic stress also causes trouble sleeping. Add that to the way we often skimp on sleep to spend more time at work or doing other things, and you have another factor that leads to meta-inflammation. When you don't get enough quality sleep, your immune function is depressed— and you know what that means.

Then there's sugar, or more accurately, high-fructose corn syrup, the form of sugar that's now found in about 90 percent of processed foods, even in products like salad dressing. Too much sugar in the diet means too much sugar in the blood, which in turn means too much of the hormone insulin in the blood, which leads to inflammation and type 2 diabetes. Excess sugar in the diet is such an important cause of inflammation that I'll discuss it in more detail later in this chapter.

Toxins

OK, I know I spent all of the last chapter talking about toxins, but I'll say it again. Your immune system sees toxins from things like cigarette smoke and air pollution as invaders to be attacked. Toxins cause inflammation.

When you have an allergic reaction, your immune system sees something that's ordinarily harmless as an invader to be destroyed. The immune response triggers inflammation. If you have hay fever, for instance, you react to pollen in the air with sneezing, a runny nose, and itchy eyes. Not all allergies are so obvious, however. Many people don't realize that they have food allergies because their reaction isn't to break out in a rash or to go into anaphylactic shock. Instead, it's often experienced as mysterious aches and pains, or digestive upsets, or leaky gut syndrome—all things that cause inflammation. One of the first things I do with new patients is go through their diet to eliminate possible allergens, such as soy and dairy foods.

When your body's pH is too low, your system is on the acidic side. Your body doesn't like that—as I discussed in Chapter 3, your body really wants to be a bit on the alkaline side. When it isn't, inflammation is one of the symptoms.

Autoimmune diseases such as fibromyalgia and chronic fatigue syndrome by definition mean you're inflamed, because your immune system is in a state of constant activation. Many of my patients with autoimmune problems really benefit from dietary approaches that reduce inflammation.

If you've got bad microbes in your body, you've got inflammation, because your immune system is turning up the heat to get rid of them. The bad microbes might be something you can overcome, like a cold virus or stomach bug, but all too often, the microbes have settled in for a long visit. A very common source of microbes is gum disease (periodontitis). The inflammation this causes isn't just seen in bleeding gums—it's generalized throughout your body. In fact, there's a strong link between gum disease and heart attacks and a range of other health issues, including premature delivery.

Your mitochondria are the tiny powerhouses in your cells that produce energy. Inflammation is both a cause and effect of damage to the mitochondria from excess oxidative stress—which comes from inflammation. When the mitochondria aren't producing at full capacity, the energy supply to your cells is reduced and they can't work as efficiently. You feel tired more than you should.

Another major cause of inflammation is methylation, or more accurately, the lack of methylation. A methyl group is a little bundle of a single carbon atom and three hydrogen atoms that normally gets attached to just about every chemical reaction that takes place in your body. The methyl group acts as a sort of on/off switch. Methylation happens constantly in your body, literally billions of times every moment. A crucial function of methylation is keeping inflammation under control. If your methylation pathways aren't working smoothly, chronic inflammation is one result.

Proper methylation needs optimal levels of all the B vitamins, but particularly folic acid (folate). Most healthy people can get enough folic acid from their food to methylate without any problems. But if you're not that healthy, or if you eat a poor diet without much in the way of fresh leafy green vegetables, you may not get enough folic acid and the other B vitamins to methylate properly. You might also have a normal genetic variant in your ability to produce an enzyme called methylene-tetra-hydro-folate-reductase, otherwise known as the MTHFR gene. If you can't produce the enzyme, you have trouble forming enough active folic acid from your food, even if you eat a diet rich in folate-containing foods. Not enough folate means poor methylation, which means inflammation. The fix for this is supplements of methylated folic acid. But because you can't know if your MTHFR gene works well or not without an expensive genetic test, I recommend to all my patients taking these supplements as a precaution.

Processed Food and Poor Posture

Ultraprocessed foods are a huge part of the Standard American Diet and a huge reason why people suffer from chronic inflammation. Researchers define these foods as "industrial formulations which, besides salt, sugar, oils and fats, include substances not used in culinary preparations. These substances include flavorings, colorings, sweeteners, and other additives that improve sensorial qualities, such as emulsifiers." These products are edible—in fact, they're engineered to be extremely tasty, even addictive—but they're not really food. They're calorie and chemical delivery mechanisms that are just really bad for your health—and they make up half of the typical American diet. When these foods are a big part of your daily diet, you're overfed but undernourished. Everything about a diet high in processed foods inflames your body even before the excess calories make you fat.

Poor posture and lack of activity are often overlooked as sources of inflammation. As a chiropractor, however, that's one of the first places I look when a patient shows signs of inflammation. I'll go into the details of why poor posture leads to inflammation in Chapter 6. For now, let's just say that it's a big downward spiral. Inflammation leads to aching muscles and joints, which leads to poor posture and lack of activity, which leads to more inflammation, which leads to even worse posture and even less activity.

SPMS: THE NATURAL ANTI-INFLAMMATORY SUPPLEMENT

We used to tell patients that inflammation just took time to go away. If you had a sprained finger, for instance, the swelling, redness, and pain would eventually go down by themselves. After the acute period passed, there wasn't much you could do to speed up the process. For a lot of patients, that's true. Their finger gradually gets back to normal over a few weeks. Sometimes, however, inflammation just won't go away. Your finger gets better, but it never completely heals and keeps hurting. When inflammation never really resolves, it becomes chronic.

That's where naturally occurring lipid mediators called specialized pro-resolving mediators (SPMs) come in. Your body naturally produces SPMs from omega-3 fatty acids as part of the resolution response to inflammation. You start to make them when the initial immune response has served its purpose. They basically tell the immune system to stop actively responding and instead to accelerate the return to homeostasis. SPMs play a unique role in helping the body finally shut down the immune response, inhibit additional inflammation, clear away the damaging byproducts of the inflammatory process, and aid tissue remodeling. Once the SPMs have done their job, the body naturally breaks them down and eliminates them.

In functional nutrition, we often recommend EPA and DHA from fish oil to help relieve inflammation. They work by competing with pro-inflammatory omega-6 fatty acids metabolites and blocking their activity. Recent research shows us this isn't the whole story. In fact, fish oil probably helps relieve inflammation the most by providing the raw material to build SPMs. The conversion process from fish oil to SPMs is complex, slow, and inefficient, even in very healthy people. In people who aren't in such great health, it's even slower. And normal genetic variation means that some people will convert even more slowly than average.

If you're healthy, you're able to produce enough SPMs to resolve the inflammation from a minor injury or illness. But what about more serious or ongoing inflammation? What about people with suboptimum health? That's when the body just can't produce enough SPMs fast enough to bring down the inflammation completely. Healing stalls out, and the protective effect of inflammation becomes destructive instead.

I'm a huge believer in making lifestyle and dietary changes to help with inflammation. And I still recommend DHA and EPA for reducing inflammation. But in more serious cases, especially when resolving the inflammation seems to be stuck, I recommend taking SPMs supplements. They're extremely effective for cases where lingering inflammation is causing ongoing pain and disability.

Right now, the only available SPMs supplement is OmegaGenics SPM Active from Metagenics. These supplements are made from fish oil using a patented fractionation process to create a SPMs-enriched product. Recent research has shown that daily dosing with two to six soft gels over six weeks produces reductions in standard inflammation blood markers such as hs-CRP, interleukins, fibrinogen, and TNF-alpha.

One really great aspect of SPMs is that because you

make them anyway as a normal part of resolving inflammation, the supplements don't suppress immunity. This makes them much safer than anti-inflammatory drugs such as glucocorticoids or methotrexate or even aspirin. SPMs supplements can be taken indefinitely. They have no known side effects or interactions with other supplements or drugs.

My usual dosing for SPMs is two capsules three times daily for during the acute inflammation stage. As inflammation becomes subacute, the dosage can be reduced to two capsules twice daily. For ongoing mild inflammation and for maintenance, I suggest two capsules once daily.

INFLAMMATION AND OBESITY

I once had a patient with 43 percent body fat. To put that in perspective, someone who's normal weight would have about 15 to 20 percent body fat. He came to me for back pain, but his true problem was the same problem all overweight people have—inflammation. Because he was so overweight, he was inflamed far more than normal. His knees were very arthritic, for example, because for every pound you're overweight you're putting four times the strain on your knee joints. Arthritis equals inflammation.

I was able to help this patient with his back pain through chiropractic treatments, but his whole system was on fire. I explained to him that his excess weight wasn't just the cause of his back pain, but it was the cause of everything else that was wrong with him as well—his headaches, his digestive problems, his mood swings—but not for the reasons he thought. I explained that his body was on fire, that we needed to put it out, and that his excess fat was the root cause.

Even if you're just a little overweight, chances are very good that you're also inflamed. That's because excess body fat, especially the kind you carry around in your waist, is actually a source of inflammation. I call it "sick fat." What's happening is that your fat cells don't just sit there storing fat—they're metabolically active, and not in a good way.

First, when you gain weight, your body stores excess energy in the form of fat mostly by stuffing it into your existing fat cells and also growing some new ones. After a point, your fat cells just can't hold any more, so you end up with extra fat circulating in your bloodstream, looking for a place to go. It often ends up being stored in places it shouldn't be, like in your liver and heart.

In your belly fat, the cells can get so large that they outstrip their blood supply. Lack of oxygen damages or even kills the cells. Damaged and dead cells trigger the immune system to come in and clean up the mess. What does that mean? Inflammation.

Fat cells also creates a lot of cytokines, hormones, and other chemical messengers that trigger inflammation. Cytokine production from fat cells may be the main reason overweight and obese people have chronic inflammation. And chronic inflammation is what causes coronary artery disease, heart attacks, and strokes. All the chemical signals sent out by fat cells create a lot of cross talk in your body. The inflammatory signals from fat cells can end up interfering with all the other chemical messengers, such as insulin, and keeping them from getting through.

BLOOD SUGAR AND INFLAMMATION

The average American eats twenty-nine pounds of French fries, twenty-three pounds of pizza, and twenty-four pounds of ice cream each year. When that diet is topped off with fifty-three gallons of soda each year, it's easy to see how someone can consume about 150 pounds of sugar and other sweeteners each year. Think of it this way: If you're an average woman, you're eating your own body weight or more in sugar each year.

According to the Department of Health and Human Services, the average American adult today gets about 13 percent of their total daily calories from sugar and added sugars. About 70 percent of people in the United States consume added sugar above the recommended limit of 10 percent of daily calories (about 10 teaspoons)—most eat the equivalent of twenty-two teaspoons of sugar every day. In the typical US diet, 31 percent of calories from added sugars come from snacks and sweets, and 47 percent come from added sugars in beverages (not including milk or 100 percent fruit juices). One-quarter of added sugars come from drinking sweetened soda.

When you eat that much sugar, you get fat. There's no other way to put it. The obesity rate in the United States is already about 35 percent. At the rate we're going, half of all Americans will be obese by 2030. And when you get fat from eating a lot of sugar, you get inflamed. Obesity has to be seen as a form of chronic low-grade inflammation.

And when you get inflamed because you're fat, you will almost certainly develop prediabetes or type 2 diabetes, along with an increased risk of arthritis, heart disease, high blood pressure, stroke, and cancer. Your chances of back problems and of needing a joint replacement sky-rocket. Today, almost 30 million Americans have type 2 diabetes—more than 9 percent of the population. Of those, about 9 million have diabetes and don't know it. They're likely to find out only when they end up in the emergency room with a heart attack. The numbers for diabetes are already bad enough, but they're projected to get worse in the coming decades.

When your body is so inflamed that you've developed type 2 diabetes, the standard medical treatment is to give you drugs that make your poor, tired pancreas squeeze out a bit more insulin and make your cells be a bit more responsive to it. You'll also be given drugs to treat everything that goes along with diabetes, like high blood pressure and high cholesterol. You'll be told to lose weight and watch out for sweets. In other words, you'll be treated from the outside in, instead of from the inside out.

A good example is how you'll be told to lose weight by cutting calories. This approach to weight loss rarely—if ever—works. Why? Because every mechanism in your body is designed to hold on to every calorie for dear life. Until very recently, the biggest problem humans ever faced was getting enough calories to survive, let alone getting fat. Our bodies simply aren't meant to deal with an excess of cheap, tasty calories all the time. Instead, we have compensatory mechanisms that defend us against weight loss by decreasing energy expenditure and increasing appetite.

When you eat a diet high in sugar and processed carbohydrates like snack foods, you're getting calories without nutrition. These foods hit your bloodstream very quickly because they take very little digestion—there's no fiber to slow their absorption. Your blood sugar spikes up. To compensate, your pancreas pours out more insulin, the hormone that carries blood sugar into your cells to be burned as energy. If the cells are full, insulin carries off the excess sugar to be stored as fat. After years of socking your pancreas with demands for insulin and gaining weight, your body starts to resist. The cells stop being as responsive to insulin—now you have insulin resistance. Your blood sugar goes up to unhealthy, inflammatory levels because it has nowhere to go. You have prediabetes or actual type 2 diabetes, depending on how far along you are in the inflammatory process. And after even more years of shocking your body with sugar, your pancreas gives up. It's so worn out that it doesn't produce enough insulin anymore. Now you need to inject insulin to survive.

All that extra sugar sloshing around in your bloodstream is doing a lot of damage. Among other things, it clogs the tiny blood vessels that nourish your eyes, your heart, and your kidneys, damaging them and setting the stage for big problems, like blindness, down the line. People with type 2 diabetes are more likely to get Alzheimer's disease as they age.

FIXING FOOD INFLAMMATION

Part of the solution to inflammation from obesity and diabetes is a diet that helps reduce inflammation. What does that mean?

- Eliminate sugar and foods with added sugar.
- Eliminate processed carbohydrates.
- Increase your intake of fresh fruits and vegetables.
- Increase your intake of fatty fish such as salmon.
- Avoid foods with gluten.
- Avoid foods with soy.
- Avoid dairy products.
- Avoid fried foods.
- Avoid foods you are sensitive to.
- Reduce or eliminate alcohol.

For severe cases, especially diabetes that's not responding well to dietary changes, I recommend a medical food called Ultra Glucose Control. This is a meal-replacement product from Metagenics that's designed to help with the nutritional management of your glucose response. It's got a balanced ratio of carbohydrates, fats, and proteins that are in line with the latest research recommendations. The complex carbohydrates in Ultra Glucose Control are released slowly into the bloodstream to help avoid glucose and insulin spikes. The powder is stirred into water as a meal replacement that helps you feel full. It also contains twenty-two essential vitamins and minerals to support overall health and monounsaturated fats to support healthy blood lipid levels. The formula helps overcome insulin resistance.

What else can you do? Sleep more, reduce stress, and get more exercise—I'll go into all of this in more detail in the next chapter.

Sugar Addiction

I can say you should cut sugar out of your diet, but that can be very hard to do. Sugar acts on the same reward centers in your brain as cocaine. You don't get addicted to it in the same way, and cutting sugar from your diet doesn't lead to withdrawal, but it's still very difficult.

Many of my patients are clearly addicted to sugar. They get a jolt of energy and a mood boost from it, but then they get a low as their blood sugar drops back down or even goes too low. That makes them crave another jolt of sugar and processed carbs.

What we want to do is modulate the jump in blood sugar and prevent the dip. In other words, we want to get the blood sugar back in balance, so it doesn't zoom too high and drop too low. The best way to do that is just to cut out the sugar altogether. To help my patients wean themselves off sugar, I recommend using stevia, a natural sweetener that is much sweeter than sugar, or a very small amount of pure maple syrup. They give the touch of sweetness that takes the edge off. Trust me, after just a couple of days of cutting sugar, you'll feel a lot better. Also, sugary foods that once tasted great will now taste unbearably sweet.

What I really don't recommend is using artificial sweeteners to replace natural sugar. These substances, such as saccharin, sucralose (Splenda), and aspartame (NutraSweet), disrupt your body's normal blood sugar controls. They alter your microbiome and impair your glucose metabolism. A lot of research tells us that people who substitute artificially sweetened soda for regular soda actually gain weight. One reason is that the sweet taste tells your body to expect calories that then it doesn't receive. Your body starts to produce insulin to deal with the sugar, but then the insulin has nothing to do—except carry sugar off to be stored as fat, thereby causing further inflammation.

If you have a leaky gut, chances are you also have a leaky brain. You're producing all sorts of cytokines, peptides, and other chemical messengers that lead to inflammation. These cross the blood-brain barrier and activate the microglia in the brain. The microglia are your brain's waste disposal system, the equivalent of macrophages (white blood cells that eat invaders). When the microglia are activated beyond normal, then you're getting inflammation and neurodegeneration in the brain. The result is short-term memory problems, brain fog, headaches, difficulty concentrating, depression, and in the long run dementia and Alzheimer's disease.

DEPRESSION AND INFLAMMATION

• • • • • •

People who are badly depressed also tend to have high blood markers for inflammation. Which comes first, depression or inflammation? Is there even a link? Recent research suggests that the brains of patients suffering from depressive episodes may be significantly inflamed—and the more severe the depression, the greater the inflammation. We still don't know if inflammation causes the depression, or is a result of it, but this research opens up promising new ways to treat a common problem.

Leaky gut syndrome and unbalanced gut bacteria are major sources of inflammation—remember, 70 percent of your immune system is in your gut. By fixing a leaky gut and getting your microbiome back in balance, as I've explained in earlier chapters, you can reduce your overall inflammation level by a *lot*. Another thing that helps reduce gut inflammation is avoiding NSAIDs such as aspirin, ibuprofen (Advil), and acetaminophen (Tylenol). Aspirin and ibuprofen are great for relieving some symptoms of inflammation, particularly pain, but in the long run they interfere with healing the source of the pain while also causing gut damage. Acetaminophen is very harmful to the liver; I recommend against it.

For severe cases of chronic inflammation, I recommend the medical food UltraInflamX Plus 360°. This is a meal-replacement powder from Metagenics that's designed to help with the nutritional management of compromised gut function. It's got a special blend of pea and rice protein, along with essential amino acids, that give you excellent nutrition—almost everyone can easily digest proteins from these sources. In addition, the blend contains key micronutrients such as folate, vitamin B12, and vitamin D, along with six grams of fiber per serving. The fats are designed to be easily absorbed and help reduce inflammation. The mix also contains glutamine, an amino acid that helps heal damaged intestines; curcumin (a natural anti-inflammatory); and selective kinase response modulators (SKRMs) that help with inflammation. I like this product because it contains targeted active ingredients that tackle gut inflammation from a lot of different angles.

PROTOCOL FOR REDUCING INFLAMMATION

For patients with severe inflammation, my 30-day protocol involves several steps.

We start with UltraInflamX Plus 360°, two scoops mixed with water twice a day. In addition, I ask the patient to take two to four grams a day of omega-3 fatty acids in the form of fish oil capsules. I also add probiotics and prebiotics.

The most important step is an anti-inflammatory diet (see the sidebar). That means no sugar or processed foods but plenty of fresh fruits and vegetables, fermented foods like sauerkraut, nuts and seeds, and berries. Just as important is avoiding irritating foods, like dairy, gluten, or soy. I individualize the diet for each patient, based on their needs and preferences and even their budget.

Diet is crucial for reducing inflammation, but other therapeutic lifestyle changes are also needed. That means exercise, supplements, and stress reduction—all topics I'll discuss later in this book. For now, it's important to remember that lifestyle changes are just as important as diet.

How do we know the protocol is working? I use standard blood tests to look for inflammation at the start of the protocol, and then check again after a month to see if there's any improvement. Among other blood markers, I look at A1C, which is a measure of blood sugar over a three-month period, and I also look at the lipid panel to see cholesterol levels. I look at several inflammatory markers, including hs-CRP, sedimentation rate, tumor necrosis factor, and interleukins. After the first month, we almost always see some improvement in everything. The lab work also tells me what's not working as well as it could and points us in the direction of additional changes. After the first month, we check the markers again every three months to make sure we're still on track and continuing to show improvement. In three months, I often see really positive changes compared to the starting point.

Reducing inflammation helps my patients in every way. They feel better in general. Their energy levels really go up, their aches and pains get better, they feel sharper, and they lose some weight even though they're not dieting. Functional nutrition works, but it does take some time. At the end of the first three months, my patients often tell me they can't believe how much better they feel.

ANTI-INFLAMMATORY DIET

. . . . . .

Fruits

Unsweetened fresh, frozen, water-packed, or canned (choose BPA-free cans); all unsweetened 100 percent fruit juice except orange juice

Avoid: Oranges

Vegetables

All fresh raw, steamed, lightly sautéed, juiced, and roasted vegetables

Avoid: Corn and creamed vegetables

Carbohydrates

Amaranth, buckwheat, millet, oats, quinoa, rice, tapioca, teff

Avoid: barley, corn, kamut, rye, spelt, wheat, all products containing gluten

Bread and Cereal

Food made from amaranth, arrowroot, buckwheat, millet, oats, potato flour, quinoa, rice, tapioca

Avoid: Foods made from barley, kamut, rye, spelt, wheat, all products containing gluten

Legumes

All beans, peas, and lentils

Avoid: soybeans, tofu, tempeh, soy milk, and other soy products

Nuts and Seeds

Almonds, cashews, pumpkin, sesame, sunflower, walnut, almond butter, cashew butter

Avoid: Peanuts, peanut butter

Meat and Fish

All BPA-free canned (water-packed), frozen, and fresh fish; chicken, turkey, lamb, venison, bison

Avoid: beef, pork, cold cuts, sausages, canned meats, eggs, shellfish

Dairy and Milk Substitutes

Milk substitutes such as almond milk, coconut milk, oat milk, rice milk, other nut milks

Avoid: Milk, cream, cheese, cottage cheese, butter, yogurt, ice cream, frozen yogurt, artificial creamers

Fats

Cold-pressed oils: almond, coconut, flax, macadamia nut, extra-virgin olive, pumpkin, walnut

Avoid: Butter, margarine, mayonnaise, shortening, processed oils, spreads

Beverages

Filtered or distilled water, herbal teas, seltzer, mineral water

Avoid: Soda, soft drinks, alcohol, coffee, tea, caffeinated beverages, sports drinks

Spices and Condiments

All spices, such as cinnamon, dill, oregano, garlic, ginger, thyme

Avoid: Chocolate, ketchup, mustard, relish, chutney, soy sauce, barbecue sauce, hot sauce

Sweeteners

Brown rice syrup, blackstrap molasses, stevia, organic maple syrup

Avoid: white sugar, brown sugar, honey, corn syrup, high-fructose corn syrup, candy, sweet desserts

Weight...Don't Tell Me!

I give a lot of talks to colleagues and to people concerned about their health. When it's time to discuss weight and nutrition, I just cut to the chase and say, "Diets don't work." That usually gets the audience's attention, because what they all really want to hear is that I've come up with some sort of super-diet that does work. But diets don't work. Most diets are simply fads. You do a juice fast, or you eliminate some specific foods, or you eat like someone who lived ten thousand years ago. You might lose some weight if you stick with it, but in the long run—like just about everyone else who has ever gone on a diet—you will go off. It's simply too hard to live with so many dietary restrictions. You'll gain back the weight you lost, and probably some additional weight as well.

Americans go on all sorts of diets all the time. The weight-loss industry is estimated to take in $64 billion a year in the United States. Despite all that money spent on dieting, today we're heavier than ever. 70 percent of all adults are overweight or obese. It's pretty clear to me that diets don't work.

What does? Quality foundational nutrition and therapeutic lifestyle changes.

DR. ROBISM

If it comes from a plant, eat it; if it's made in a plant, don't!

DR. ROBISM

Not all calories are created equal. You could fit a lot of broccoli into the same thousand calories as a frappucino.

DR. ROBISM

I prescribe a new weight-loss drug to my patients. It's a forkful of green vegetables.

THE DIET THAT WORKS

· · · · · ·

There's one diet that does work, but it's not for losing weight—it's to keep you from losing your mind to dementia and Alzheimer's disease. Developed by researchers at the Rush University Medical Center, it's called the MIND diet, short for Mediterranean-DASH Intervention for Neurodegenerative Delay. The diet can lower the risk of Alzheimer's by as much as 53 percent if you really stick to it and by about 35 percent if you follow it only moderately well. The MIND diet is a hybrid of the Mediterranean and DASH (Dietary Approaches to Stop Hypertension) diets, both of which have been found to reduce the risk of hypertension, heart attack, and stroke.

The MIND diet has fifteen dietary components, including ten that are well-known to be brain-healthy: leafy green vegetables, other vegetables, nuts, berries, beans, whole grains, fish, poultry, olive oil, and wine. The five foods to avoid are red meat, butter and margarine, cheese, pastries and sweets, and fried or fast food.

DON'T DIET

Lots of my patients have tried every diet that has come along. They've discovered that none work for long-term weight loss, and all left them worse off. They don't want to try yet another fad diet, so they come to me to learn about healthy eating, not dieting.

When we talk about what healthy foods are, I often encounter a lot of resistance based on cost. I want my patients to choose organic products and avoid cheap processed foods. Real food is more expensive on the surface, but when you start eating it, you realize that you're actually saving money. That's because when you compare the cost of calories to nutrients, or calories to feeling satisfied, or calories to health, a healthy diet of real food is really much cheaper. Compare the cost of an organic apple to a can of soda. It takes two apples to equal the 120 calories in the soda. The apples cost about fifty cents apiece; the soda costs over a dollar. So, for the same dollar and the same calories, you can eat two apples or drink one soda. The apples are nice and crunchy, they're naturally sweet, they're full of fiber, and they're a great source of vitamin C, potassium, and phytonutrients. There's no nutrition whatsoever in the soda. After eating two apples, you feel full and won't be hungry for a while. The soda can actually make you feel hungrier because diet soda messes with your blood sugar. Dollar for dollar, the apples are a bargain.

Diets don't work because they're too restrictive. I believe that you shouldn't go on a diet that you can't sustain for a lifetime. That means you shouldn't go on a diet at all, because none of them are truly sustainable. They're all based on faulty thinking. Take the HCG diet, for instance. It's based on the idea that by going on an ultra-low-calorie diet—just five hundred calories a day— and taking supplements of human chorionic gonadotropin (the HCG part). you'll lose a lot of weight, supposedly up to a pound a day. You'll also magically "reset" your metabolism without feeling hungry, tired, or sick.

This is a great example of why diets don't work and can even be harmful—the only thing that will really get lighter will be your wallet. You can't sustain five hundred calories a day for long. You're starving yourself and not getting the protein and other nutrients you need for normal metabolism. You're also putting incredible stress on your liver—check back to Chapter 3 on toxins to see why. You lose weight on the HCG diet because you're getting so few calories. The HCG shots and supplements (not approved by the FDA, by the way) supposedly let you eat a very low-calorie diet by suppressing your appetite and keeping you from losing muscle.

If you restrict your calories on any sort of diet, you'll lose weight—at first. Then your body's natural compensatory mechanisms will kick in, and your weight loss will slow or even stop. Cutting calories further will only make your body even more eager to hang on to every last calorie it can, because it thinks you're living in a famine environment. At the same time, the calorie hypothesis is flawed, because so many other factors regulate your metabolism. There's the dietary composition of your food, but there's also your toxic load, your food allergies and sensitivities, any drugs you have to take, your overall health, your hormones, and even who your friends are.

I've seen patients try the HCG diet—and every other fad diet, like juice fasts and the paleo diet. After a while, they give up on whatever the diet is and come to me to undo the damage and get them back on track with eating real food in sustainable amounts.

The model of "going on a diet" is just wrong. My patients think of dieting as a jail term. They feel deprived and restricted, to say nothing of being hungry, all the time. Even when I help them change their diet so that they lose weight while learning to eat in a sustainable and healthy way, they ask me, "When can I go off this?" I reply, "Why would you want to stop watching what you're eating? Why would you all of a sudden want to get unhealthy again?" When they see it that way, they stop seeing the changes in their eating habits as a diet and start seeing the changes as a permanent, healthy lifestyle.

The true reason for getting fat isn't overeating. It's the opposite: Being fat leads to overeating and getting fatter and sicker. That's because when you're overweight, your fat cells are stuffed with stored fat and accumulated toxins. As I explained back in Chapter 4, that leads to inflammation, which causes, among other things, high levels of insulin in your blood. A major function of insulin is to store excess blood sugar as fat—and so the cycle of getting fatter goes on. Your body sucks up your calories to store them as fat. That makes your brain think you actually aren't getting enough to eat, so it makes you want to eat more, while also slowing your metabolism to conserve energy.

Right now we have lots of different diets, but no one

has a lifestyle. None of these diets are working. If they were, we wouldn't have a constantly increasing obesity rate. Losing weight is a classic example of a problem that needs to be treated from the inside out. The answer isn't counting calories—it's improving the quality of what you eat.

CHANGE WHAT YOU EAT

To lose weight permanently in a healthy way, you've got to change what you eat, not necessarily how much you eat. All calories aren't created equal.

The conventional diet approach is calories in, calories out. Eat fewer calories, and you'll lose weight. But that's not really true. It's not how many calories you eat, it's where they come from. If you want to eat 1,000 calories, you could eat twenty Oreos (fifty calories per cookie), or you could eat nearly three pounds of cooked kale. It's all too easy to imagine eating twenty Oreos over the course of a day, but eating three pounds of kale would take some commitment. It's not the calories; it's the nutrients. You'll get a lot more nutrition from a real food like kale than from a manufactured food like Oreos.

DR. ROBISM

When a patient tells me she drinks socially, I ask, "Well, how social are you? Are you social every night? Are you social once a week?"

The other key to weight loss is portion control. Today we have a lot of portion distortion. We've been supersizing our portions for so long that they seem normal to us now. All that means is larger portions of junkier food. We simply eat too much at every meal and snack. When something is called family-sized, it means it's supposed to feed a family, not one person. Ever since the food government dietary guidelines were issued back in 1971, we've been encouraged to avoid dietary fat and eat carbohydrates. Soon after, cheap high-fructose corn syrup started to be widely used, so fast food restaurants could supersize your soda and still make money. We can look back and date the start of the obesity epidemic to that time. We can also date the reality that obesity takes eight years off your life, and destroys your quality of life before that, back to the 1970s. Since then, obesity has become a worldwide problem. No nation has yet succeeded in lowering or even slowing their national obesity rates.

Today, it's hard to escape food. Go to a staff meeting, and donuts are on the conference table. Every receptionist has a candy dish on the desk. How can you turn down birthday cake or homemade Christmas cookies? If everyone else on the sales team is going out for pizza, you have to go as well.

Lots of people tell me that they can't help being overweight, because it's in their genes. They just have a "heavy build," so trying to lose weight is pointless. It's true that genes can account for about 10 to 30 percent of obesity, but you're not a prisoner of your genes—plus even 30 percent isn't that substantial. Our genes haven't changed, but our environment has. Study after study has shown lifestyle changes can lead to long-term weight control.

The primary driver of chronic disease is the interaction between your genes, your activities of daily living, and your environment. There's an old saying in health care: Genes load the gun, but environment pulls the trigger. You may have inherited some genes that make you tend to gain weight, but if your food and lifestyle environment are healthy, that obesity bullet may never get fired.

Sometimes a patient says to me, "My mom was fat, my father was fat, and I'm fat. I'm just stuck with fat genes." Really? Think of it this way: Lots of people have reached the highest levels of education even when neither one of their parents finished high school. It's the same thing with weight. You can tap your own potential to be healthy. I always say, "Be stretched by your goals. Don't be inhibited by your excuses."

DR. ROBISM

Exercise is good for you, but you can't outrun a bad diet.

DETOXING FOR WEIGHT LOSS

Changing your diet and your lifestyle are key to weight

loss, but there's one more step that needs to be taken at the start. You need to detox.

Your fat cells are where a lot of toxins, like the BPA we talked about in Chapter 4, end up being stored. Most chemical toxins are fat-soluble. The more fat cells you have, the more toxins you're storing. That can make weight loss very difficult.

Here's the scenario I see with a lot of my patients. They need to lose thirty pounds, so they start to cut calories. They eat nothing but baked chicken, brown rice, and broccoli and add in some exercise. Everything goes great for the first ten pounds or so, and then the weight loss stops. They hit a plateau, so they cut back on calories even more and spend more time on the treadmill. They stay stuck on the plateau and get so frustrated that they just stop trying to lose weight.

What's really happening is that their body's fat-burning process has stopped because shrinking their fat cells means less storage space for the toxins. The toxins get released into the body and cause inflammation. The body slows down its metabolism because it doesn't want to make itself sick by trying to cope with all those toxins at once. At the same time, the liver is struggling to rid them of this sudden flood of toxins into the bloodstream.

To lose weight safely, I strongly recommend doing a ten-day detox to keep your metabolism from slowing down and keeping you from shedding pounds. Repeat the detox if your weight loss slows, and do it again when you reach your goal weight. After that, detox regularly, every spring and fall.

QUALITY FOUNDATIONAL NUTRITION

Quality foundational nutrition is very simple: Eat real, unprocessed foods, preferably organic. The rule of thumb is to eat foods that have been minimally changed from their natural state. It's the difference between an organic baked potato and a plastic dish containing microwaved frozen scalloped potatoes. The baked potato is a whole food, while potato isn't even the first ingredient on the label for the scalloped potatoes. OK, I agree that those scalloped potatoes taste great. They've been engineered to seduce your taste buds with salt, additive, high-fructose corn syrup, and bad fats. One of my patients once told me, "I got 1600 on my SATs, but I can't understand what all those ingredients on the food labels are." I told him not to bother trying to understand—just skip those foods instead. I don't see any food labels on fruits and vegetables, whole grains, organic beef, fish, and other healthy foods.

My patients often want me to "prescribe" a diet for them. I do often prescribe medical foods for people with serious inflammation or blood sugar problems, but for most patients, I work with them to individualize their diet based on the concept of quality foundational nutrition.

We work out an eating plan they can live with comfortably, without hunger, and that still lets them eat their favorite foods.

What's just as important is helping them understand portion control. When it comes to broccoli, you can eat all you want, but you can't do that with most foods. Portion control sounds restrictive, but it really isn't. We know that if you give someone a lot of a food, they'll eat it just because it's in front of them, not because they're really hungry or even particularly enjoy the food. Portion control helps people realize that they can feel satisfied by much smaller portions than they usually eat. I don't want my patients counting calories or fat grams. I don't want them to mess around with scales and measuring out their food. Instead, I teach them to use visual ways to estimate their portions. Some examples are as follows:

- 3.5 ounces of fish, chicken, or meat are about the size of a deck of cards or a bar of soap.
- 6 ounces of fish, chicken, or meat are about the size of a thin paperback book.
- 1 cup of berries is about the size of a baseball.
- 2 tablespoons of nut butter are about the size of a golf ball.
- 1 cup of rice or vegetables is about the size of a baseball.

Another way to look at portions is to compare them to your hand. Here's the idea:

- 1/2 cup of cooked pasta is about the size of the front of your clenched fist.
- 3.5 ounces of fish, chicken, or meat are about the size of your palm.
- 1 cup of anything (rice, vegetables, breakfast cereal) is about the size of your clenched fist.

NUTRITIONAL SUPPLEMENTS

After years of unhealthy dieting, many of my patients need supplements to improve their basic nutritional status. When your cells are depleted of nutrients, food alone, no matter how nutrient-rich it is, can never replete them—you need supplements to restore high nutrient levels in your cells. I tailor the supplements to each patient, but I almost always include a complete multivitamin with minerals supplement along with fish oil, extra vitamin D, and a green drink. Once my patients are back on a good nutritional path, I want them getting their vitamins, minerals, phytonutrients, and everything else from their food, not supplements. The cost of supplements can add up—I'd rather see you spend that money on good, nutrient-dense foods instead.

I ask my patients to buy only supplements that have been certified by a reputable third party. The product label should say something about third-party certification. If it doesn't, don't buy the product. Third-party certification guarantees that what's on the label is in the bottle—and that the product doesn't contain any undeclared ingredients, like artificial colors or gluten. The third party is usually a lab that provides independent testing to evaluate supplements and their ingredients. The other thing to look for on the label is a statement saying that the product was made according to good manufacturing processes (GMP). Again, if you can't find that on the label, don't buy the product.

If you feel you need supplements in addition to your basic food, I recommend working with a professional to decide what you need and why. Just reading an article about the latest hot supplement isn't a good way to decide what's best for you.

I'm a big proponent of medical foods for patients with serious problems related to inflammation and blood sugar. Medical foods are foods that are specially formulated and intended for the dietary management of disease. They're supplements for people with distinct nutritional needs that can't be met by a normal diet alone. If, for instance, you would really benefit from the anti-inflammatory phytonutrients found in cruciferous vegetables like broccoli and kale, you won't be able to eat enough of these foods to provide what you need. That's where a medical food or green drink can be very helpful.

Here's my list of top supplements for weight loss:

- A medical food for weight loss: I use the UltraMeal Plus 360 from Metagenics for my patients because it has targeted, quality nutrients, improves insulin sensitivity, and is very low on the glycemic index, so it doesn't spike blood sugar.

- Fish oil: I prefer the OmegaGenics® EPA-DHA 720 product from Metagenics. It contains a good balance of the essential fatty acids EPA (eicosapentaenoic acid) and DHA (docosahexaenoic acid), made from high-quality fish oil. This supplement is helpful for improving body composition.

- Vitamin D3 in the form of cholecalciferol. Most overweight people are low in vitamin D.

- Probiotics, as explained in Chapter 1.

- Conjugated linoleic acid (CLA): CLA is a fatty acid found naturally in dairy foods and meat. It can help with weight loss by helping you retain lean muscle mass and lose only fat. It also helps control type 2 diabetes. Researchers still don't know exactly how it works, but I have seen very good results with my patients. It seems to help with losing love handles and excess fat in the hip area.

- Alpha lipoic acid (ALA): Alpha-lipoic acid is a powerful antioxidant and helps protect against cell damage. It's helpful for stabilizing blood sugar and for improving cell membrane health.

Your weight alone doesn't tell you much about your body. Serious athletes are often heavier than normal for their height and sex, because they carry a lot of muscle. You could be within the normal weight range for your height and sex and turn out to have a lot of body fat.

Ideally, a normal healthy man has between 14 and 18 percent body fat; a normal healthy woman has between 21 and 24 percent body fat. In men, a body fat percentage of 26+ means obesity; in women, it's 32+. When you lose weight, you don't want to just weigh less. You also want to have a better ratio of body fat to muscle. If that doesn't happen, you can lose weight but not see any improvement in performance. You won't get through your activities of daily living any better, for example. And because the more muscle you have, the better your body deals with aging, it's important to build and maintain muscle mass.

I like to evaluate the body composition of my patients on a regular basis. This is very easy to do with the InBody body composition analyzer in my office. This is a machine that looks a bit like the scale in the doctor's office but with arms. It weighs you and also measures your body fat using bioelectrical impedance analysis. It gives me a very accurate picture of how much fat and how much muscle you have. Based on your body composition, I can say you're a strong heavy person or you're a weak light person.

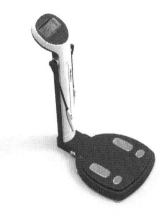

One of the things I like about the InBody is that it analyzes how your body changes with better nutrition. You might not be losing weight by the scale, but the InBody shows you that, while your weight has remained the same, your body composition has improved. The InBody machine divides the body up into five areas, so you can really understand your body composition. It gives you a detailed picture of your body composition in each arm, each leg, and your trunk. You can easily see any imbalances that way.

Another great thing about the InBody is that it shows you where your fat is. It can show that you have a lot of visceral fat—the fat that's stored inside your abdominal area, packed around your important internal organs. It also shows where your subcutaneous fat—the fat under your skin—lies. You can pinch your subcutaneous fat, but not your visceral fat.

Visceral fat is especially dangerous for causing inflammation and heart disease. We know that diet plus exercise helps you lose subcutaneous fat. We also know that exercise doesn't really help you lose visceral fat, so you really need to focus on diet.

I like to see body composition of about 15 percent or less fat for men and about 22 percent fat for most women. If you keep your body composition in an optimum range, you're definitely going to have a better posture and a better movement pattern, because you're not straining your body.

When I first meet with a new patient who wants to lose weight, we do a health assessment and a nutritional assessment. I want to know the patient's medical history, including what medications they're taking and what health conditions they have. The health appraisal questionnaire asks about ten different systems in the body, with numbers ranking their health. The higher the number, the more complaints the patient has. Some of my patients come in at a rank of sixty, which is rather high. After we make dietary and lifestyle changes, the health appraisal number often drops to thirty just a month later.

In the nutritional survey, I ask how often the patient has dieted in the past and what diet they followed. We also do a review of what they ate over the past three to seven days. I ask if they think they ate a healthy diet during that time. Patients often think they did, even when they obviously didn't. A big part of what I do is simply educate my patients about what true healthy eating means. Finally, and most importantly, I ask the patients what their goals are. We want to have a clear, realistic idea of what we want to accomplish. That helps us plan additional therapeutic lifestyle changes that will be attainable and successful.

My goal is to have my patients no longer ask me what they should eat. I want to educate them to the point where they know what's good for them and no longer need to follow a diet plan or food list. They can then make informed and educated decisions on their own about what to eat.

As part of the initial assessment, I do blood work to get baseline numbers for things like cholesterol, blood sugar, inflammation markers, and pH.

I use the health assessment, the nutritional assessment, and the body composition information to get an inside-out picture of the body.

THIRTY-DAY KICK START

I get my patients moving toward better health with a thirty-day quality foundational nutrition program I call a kick start. The program starts with a ten-day detoxification, as explained in Chapter 3. Once we've gotten the liver to function well, we can move on to a less intense ongoing detox with dietary changes that also help build up the gut—

and usually also lead to weight loss. My patients never feel they're on a diet, however, because the program isn't restrictive in terms of calories and offers a wide variety of foods. Most of my patients do well with a Mediterranean-style diet that emphasizes fresh vegetables, fruits, whole grains, fish, and very little sugar. A few patients seem to do better with, or prefer, a paleo diet that emphasizes organic meats and only some vegetables, with very few carbohydrates such as fruits or grains. This approach isn't for everyone, and I don't recommend it in the long run, but for some patients, it's a good starting point.

I also do a lot of gluten-free diets. If you're sensitive to gluten, you're also very inflamed. There's no good test for gluten sensitivity, so one way to find out is to cut gluten and see what happens. I've seen inflammation really drop in some patients when they do this. It goes right back up again if they eat gluten-containing grains such as wheat, barley, or rye.

A TYPICAL PATIENT

When I think about a typical patient, I think of a woman who is around age forty, is about thirty-five pounds overweight, and has a high body fat percentage. We do all the tests and assessments. Once I have the results, we sit down together and make a game plan that's designed just for her and her particular needs, likes, and dislikes. We take into account her health status and the drugs she has to take. We also take her daily life into account and work therapeutic lifestyle changes into it. Most importantly, we discuss her attitude. She's probably tried a lot of diets already, which means she's likely to get frustrated faster if she doesn't see improvement or if she starts to feel as if she's being deprived or sent to jail. We also discuss eating triggers. What makes her go for the ice cream or the Oreos late at night? How can we work around that? It often turns out to be a problem with low blood sugar, which makes you crave carbohydrates and sweets. We can start to fix the problem just by getting the blood sugar on a more even keel. That is often enough to cut back on the desire to snack or to avoid the late-night trigger.

My job is to motivate patients and help them stick with the program. It's also to help patients learn to be more accepting of themselves. When someone goes off the plan, I don't want them to stay off. I want them to forgive themselves and get right back to it the next day. Michael Jordan misses plenty of game-winning shots; even the best hitters in baseball only connect one out of three times. Going off the plan for a day isn't the end of the world. In my experience, if you stick with it 80 percent of the time, you'll lose weight and feel better. If you stick with it even more, then so much the better.

When the ten-day detox is over, I'll see her starting to understand what good food is and realizing that it tastes great. She'll feel better and look better—the dark rings under her eyes will start to dissipate, her skin and hair will look better, and she'll already feel and see a difference in her body composition. Most of all, she won't be feeling deprived or hungry all the time.

A lot of my patients think they're on a weight-loss program. They're not. They're on a better body composition program. It's not a diet with a beginning and an ending point. It's a therapeutic plan to change their body composition to less fat and more muscle. My patients do well on it because they lose weight and get healthy at the same time. They're dieting without dieting.

DR. ROB ISM

The only way to lose weight on the Standard American Diet is not to eat it.

DR. ROB ISM

I like what motivational speaker Jim Rohn says: "Take care of your body; it's the only place you have to live."

CASE STUDY: THE PATIENT WHO TRIED EVERYTHING
. . . . . .

A few years ago, a fifty-four-year-old woman named Evelyn came to see me. She weighed just over three hundred pounds. Her direct motivation for making the appointment was a remark she overheard when she was clothes shopping. One salesperson said to another, "She should go to the circus and buy a tent."

Evelyn told me she had tried every diet on earth. She would lose weight, then go off the diet and regain the lost weight plus twenty pounds. She was tired of yo-yo dieting, tired of weighing so much, and tired of trying to lose weight.

When I looked at her blood work, I could see she was probably the most inflamed patient I've ever had. She was also on the verge of type 2 diabetes. I called her the fire engine. The first step was to get her onto a medical food from Metagenics called Ultra Glucose Control to calm the inflammation and start healing her gut. I added probiotic, CLA, and alpha lipoic acid for her blood sugar, and started a ten-day detox. We also agreed that she would aim for ten thousand steps a day, a big improvement for her. Evelyn began to lose weight rapidly. Over three months, she lost sixty pounds as she learned to eat a quality diet. Her body composition really improved—and because she had less fat and more muscle, she was able to add some aerobic exercise and weight training to her ten thousand steps, which improved her body composition even more.

I continue to see Evelyn, but just once every three months. She knows what to do now and continues to lose weight, though more slowly. She says she feels better every time I see her. Evelyn is a lawyer, and she tells me that her weight loss and better health let her get through her long workdays much more easily—to the point where her caseload has increased. Her weight, her health, and her career have all improved. Evelyn had been down a lot of roads that turned into dead ends. For me, it was very gratifying to help her finally find the right path.

Life in Motion

For me, movement is the key. Movement tells me the story of a person's life injuries, both in the past and possibly down the road. A disturbing number of patients come to me because their movement is compromised and they're in pain. Many of my patients can't lift their arms above their shoulders. They want me to fix their problems with chiropractic techniques. I do that, but that's just the start. Because the problem comes from within, we need to take an inside-out approach to fix it.

If you don't fix the underlying injury, you're never going to get a good clinical outcome from manual therapy.

For most people, poor movement began years earlier, probably with an injury. Maybe you banged your knee, which made you limp around for a few days until the inflammation went down. You compensated for the imbalance caused by the limping by using other muscles to move. You got over the bang to your knee and forgot about it, but your body and your brain didn't. The limp made subtle, permanent differences in how you move and how your brain perceives where you are relative to everything else around you (proprioception). You're now more likely to have another injury and develop arthritis in your joints, because your movement is out of balance.

As the years and injuries accumulate, so does inflammation. Your movement gets worse. You're less flexible, you can't bend over well or raise your arms, and you have aches and pains that make you want to sit in your lounge chair instead of being active.

You might have cumulative trauma disorder from repeated injuries, like when you throw your back out in the same place more than once. Another good example of cumulative trauma disorder is carpal tunnel syndrome, where the nerve that passes through a narrow passage in your wrist gets compressed and causes pain. You might not even feel the injuries when they happen, because we're all constantly doing things to ourselves just as part of daily living. If you constantly injure yourself in the same place, though, there's insufficient tissue recovery time between the injury cycles. The tissue damage accumulates, then there's a breakdown, and then there's pain.

Most people think that if they feel no pain, then they haven't really hurt themselves, because they're below what we call the symptomatic injury threshold. They figure that if it doesn't hurt, then there's nothing wrong. Even if it doesn't hurt now, if your movement isn't good, it will hurt later on. Repetition does the real damage.

Injury occurs when the applied load is over the tissue tolerance. In other words, your back goes out when you lift something heavier than the muscles can handle. That's when you get the initial injury or cumulative trauma. When your movement patterns are unbalanced, you have poor functional performance—you're in pain, and even tying your shoes can be a problem. You're also much more likely to injure yourself. And because injury causes movement adaptation to avoid pain, you'll only get more out of balance when that happens.

HOW YOUR MUSCLES MOVE

A fundamental concept in physiology is Sherrington's Law of Reciprocal Innervation: When one set of muscles is stimulated, muscles opposing the action of the first set are simultaneously inhibited. This was first demonstrated by Sir Charles Scott Sherrington, who won the Nobel Prize in Medicine or Physiology in 1932 for his work. Sherrington was talking about your skeletal muscles, the ones you can see and feel. As you might have guessed from their name, skeletal muscles attach to the skeleton and are how you move your body. The important thing to remember is that skeletal muscles come in pairs. You need one muscle to move the joint and bone in one direction, and another to move it back.

The pain dynamic in the body is set up when you have a skeletal muscle that gets tightened or shortened from an injury or overuse. Because every muscle has a balancing muscle, the balancing muscle also gets inhibited. The brain just shuts it off. Now you have one muscle that's tight and shortened and another that's lengthened. The strain point or what I call the base of the balance is the nearest joint. That strain point leads to pain, typically pain that sends a patient to me.

You can see how this works if you do a biceps curl, where you hold a weight in your hand with your arm extended and then move the weight up and in toward your shoulder. You'll feel the large biceps muscle in your upper arm move—it's the muscle that gets big when Popeye eats his spinach. The balancing muscle to the biceps is the triceps, in the under part of your upper arm. When you do a biceps curl, the biceps muscle shortens and tightens, while the triceps muscle lengthens. As you lower the weight, the biceps stretches and the triceps shortens. Sherrington's Law applies to every muscle in your body. Every time you take a step, some muscles are tightening and some are shortening. The message telling the muscles what to do originates in the brain and is sent to the muscles by the nerves. If we want to change movement, we also need to retrain how the brain sends the messages.

POSTURE AND MOVEMENT

Sherrington said, "Posture follows movement like a shadow." I see that every day in my office. I can look at somebody's posture and see right away what injuries that person has already had and what injuries they're probably going to get. If I see you walk with your left foot turned out, running or putting weight on it will only make it worse. I can see just from the way you sit in a chair if you bend your lower back at the spine or from the hips. That tells me whether you're likely to have lower back problems (you will if you bend from the spine). I can also see how your posture and the position of your head puts stress on the vertebrae in your neck. If you hold your head in a forward position, for instance, it's like stressing your neck by putting a fifty-pound weight on it. One of the first things I work on with my patients is their posture. Not only does this improve how they feel; it improves how they appear to others. People who stand up straight and are well balanced make a better impression. That might be because standing up straight makes you produce higher levels of the neurotransmitter serotonin and lower amounts of the stress hormone cortisol.

When your body isn't in the right alignment, your body will steal stability from somewhere else in order to feel safe and not in danger of falling over. It robs strength from one part and gives it to another. We call that compensation. An injury or imbalance makes the body compensate and adapt to avoid pain. Our bodies naturally want safety and stability above all and will do anything to obtain it. You're held together by interconnecting joints that link all your muscles. To improve your functional movement, we want to look at all of you, not just some isolated muscles. Assessing how somebody moves is a powerful indicator or predictor of injury.

Among those interconnecting joints, some are mobile and some are stable. For example, your hips should be mobile, while your lumbar (lower) spine should be stable. Often, when someone has lower back pain, it's because a joint isn't as mobile as it should be. When your hips aren't mobile, you have to compensate for that somewhere—and that usually ends up meaning the lumbar spine or maybe your knee. If a joint that's supposed to be stable, like the lumbar spine, is forced to move in unnatural ways, injury ensues.

What comes first, injury or pain? It doesn't really matter. If you move poorly and that motion has been ingrained in your brain, you're going to get injured and be in pain. Ankle sprains are a great example. You limp when you sprain your ankle. It seems to heal up, but in the meantime, limping around for weeks has retrained your brain to move the ankle abnormally. Because it doesn't hurt anymore, you think your new way of walking is what's normal and that you're now walking the way you did before the sprain. Chances are you're not—and that's one of the reasons ankle sprains recur 80 percent of the time. To avoid this outcome, we need to retrain your movement. Flexibility training is particularly helpful. However, although you can train flexibility, that doesn't transfer to mobility and functional movement patterns. Training and rehab programs may benefit from an additional focus on what we call grooving new motor patterns.

To groove a new motor pattern into your brain, you have to practice the pattern. Otherwise, your brain won't remember it. Poor movement patterns exist only in the brain. So, as Yoda said, you must unlearn what you have learned. At the end of the day, to fix any movement problems, you should apply treatment, exercise, nutritional protocols, and motor control protocols to achieve positive outcomes.

PROPRIOCEPTION

Proprioception is always altered after an injury. The right muscles now aren't doing the right thing at the right time. Back injuries are a good example. If you hurt your lower back and get sent for an MRI to look at the discs between the vertebrae, they may look fine. There's no sign of damage or herniation. Then a couple of years later, your back goes out again and this time you do have herniated discs. What happened? The first injury set you up for the second. Your movement after the first injury never really returned to normal. After that, you probably started flexing your spine at the lumbar region instead of at the hips. The stress on the nerves and spinal discs made you release inflammatory cytokines, which can eat away at the cartilage and disc material in your spine. Eventually, the disc breaks down and bulges out from its normal position between two vertebrae. Recent research has shown that people with lower back pain have higher levels of an inflammation marker called interleukin-6. The higher the level, the more likely they were to have spinal stenosis and degenerative disc disease. The findings suggest that people with lower back pain have chronic low-grade inflammation.

DOCTOR ROB'S MAGNIFICENT SEVEN

Movement never lies. It tells the unique story of each individual's physical history, compensations, and adaptations. When I do a functional movement assessment, I look at seven movements, what I modestly call Doctor Rob's Magnificent Seven. The purpose of the movement assessment is to see how the body initiates and finishes movements, relative to the position that starts and stops it.

- **Movement 1.** The first movement I look at is your basic standing posture and where you feel pain. Posture pain is a definite sign that something's wrong.
- **Movement 2.** The overhead squat, a CrossFit move where you lift a barbell over your head while doing a squat. The overhead squat checks for flexion and extension in the hips, knees, and feet. It checks the strength of your core to stabilize your lower body, and it also tests your upper body flexibility. A lot of very muscular, fit guys can't get the bar over their head because they have breaks in their movement. If you can't do this move fluidly, the places where your movement is improper are where you're going to get injuries.
- **Movement 3.** The one-legged squat. Most people can't do this, even though, if you think about it, we spend more time on one leg when we walk and move than on both legs. When people can't do this movement, it's usually because they have a problem with proprioception or because they have a problem with their gluteus maximus, medius and minimus.
- **Movement 4.** The trunk stability push-up, a good way to see how strong your core is. If your core strength is good, you should be able to do this in one fluid motion, without any breaks. Planks are another good way to test for core strength.
- **Movement 5.** The valgus jump test. *Valgus* means

twisted outward from the centerline of the body (the opposite, *varus*, means twisted inward). A valgus deformity in the knees gives a knock-kneed appearance that is especially visible if you jump up and down. Knee valgus is a risk factor for injuring the anterior cruciate ligament (ACL) in the knee and also for other knee injuries, such as osteoarthritis.

- **Movement 6.** Upper/lower muscle firing patterns. This is a series of short tests used to assess muscle imbalances and faulty movement patterns. They test posture, strength, flexibility, and balance and how they work together. Firing patterns are a good way to pinpoint weak areas and correct them to avoid injury. I often say to patients, "I don't care where you go; I care how you get there." In a shoulder abduction (moving your arms up and out from the midline, like when you do a jumping jack), I'm looking at the fluidity of the movement. If you can't do this smoothly and easily, it could indicate that the rotator cuff and deltoid muscles are not firing in the right sequence. When doing a hip extension (as in doing a prone leg lift), again, I want to see if the muscle firing patterns are in the right sequence, with the gluteus maximus firing first. If you use your lower back muscles to raise your leg instead, this is setting you up for movement problems, soft-tissue injuries, and joint failure down the line.

- **Movement 7.** Regular push-up. I feel everyone should be able to do a full push-up. The push-up is a good way to evaluate upper body strength and core strength. Push-ups can be very revealing for movement pattern failures or muscle imbalance. Someone who can't go up and down all the way usually has a stability issue or a power issue, or sometimes both. For example, if the core bends during the push-up, that indicates an imbalance in the abdominal muscles.

THE EPIDEMIC OF SITTING

Because we all sit so much, we have an epidemic of bad head posture. We're always in a head-forward position—when we watch TV, sit at the computer, drive a car, or look at our smartphones. That means that your head is pushed forward in front of your shoulders, instead of balancing over them. As we spend even more time in this position, especially looking at electronic screens, it's a tsunami of ergonomic accidents and muscle imbalances waiting to happen. I call it the neuro-musculoskeletal detonation sequence. Your head is the weight of a bowling ball, about ten pounds on average. For every inch that it is pushed forward, there's an exponential increase of pressure in your neck.

A study conducted by the shoe manufacturer Reebok in 2016 showed that the average person will spend 29.75

percent of his or her life sitting down, either at work or at home, and less than 1 percent of his or her time exercising. What's the solution to the sitting epidemic? Stand up and walk around. That can help balance out the rounded shoulders and tilted pelvis we get when we hunch forward. Another important factor is losing weight. When you're carrying a beer gut or have an apple shape, that tilts your pelvis forward; you have to hunch forward and turn your feet out to compensate. If you're very heavy in the gluteus maximus and thighs, you're basically waddling instead of walking.

HOW MUCH EXERCISE DO YOU NEED?

Not everyone has to be an exercise nut like me and work out every day, but everyone has to exercise. At the lightest level, that means aiming for ten thousand steps a day. Buy a good pedometer or exercise device and work at just walking more—it can be very helpful. If you have prediabetes or type 2 diabetes, exercise is critical for keeping your blood sugar under control. I strongly recommend thirty minutes of exercise every day. Walking is a great choice.

At the highest level of exercise is weight training with barbells, but that's really not for everyone. For rehab and regular moderate workouts, I like kettlebells. These are cast-iron, ball-shaped weights with a single handle. They come in a range of sizes and weights. Instead of lifting them, as you do with dumbbells and barbells, you swing the kettlebells. The swing is great for exercising the hips; holding the handle is great for handgrip strength. Kettlebells are inexpensive to buy; you don't have to buy any other equipment to use them. You can find lots of great kettlebell exercises and workouts online, such as at dragondoor.com and strongfirst.com.

My patients always tell me that they don't have time to work out or exercise. It's the adult version of the dog ate my homework—an excuse I see right through. First of all, if you care about your long-term health, you'll find the time. Study after study show that fitness correlates with health, especially as you age. In fact, a recent study showed that the brains of older adults who exercise regularly are, in terms of function, ten years younger than people the same age who don't exercise regularly. Lots of other studies show that your "fitness age," as determined by your cardiovascular endurance, is a better predictor of longevity than your chronological age. The good news here is that unlike your actual age, you can lower your fitness age through exercise.

All you really need for your daily workout is four minutes. In that time, you can do a set of Tabata exercises (named for the Japanese trainer who developed them) that exercise your whole body and build up your endurance. In a Tabata workout, you work hard for twenty seconds, then rest for ten seconds, then repeat the cycle eight times for a total of four minutes. It's a form of high-intensity interval training, or HIIT. It's a great way to get your heart rate up and an effective alternative to traditional endurance-based training, because it causes superior physiological adaptation.

Can't you find four minutes in your day to exercise?

I have to point out that Tabata or HIIT isn't the best choice if you have any sort of chronic issue, like an arthritic knee. You need gentler exercises, like walking. Even then, however, you can do interval training. Walk as fast as you can for a few minutes, then return to your normal pace, then walk faster again. My point is that everyone can exercise, even those who have chronic health problems or painful joints. Work with your chiropractor or personal trainer to find exercises that you can do comfortably and regularly.

CORE STRENGTHENING

Your core consists of twenty-nine pairs of muscles in your trunk and pelvis. When you strengthen your core, you involve all the muscles in your lower back, pelvis, hips, and abdomen to work together. Your core muscles fall into two types: local and global. The local muscles are stability muscles; the global muscles are used for dynamic movement. If you think of your spinal cord as the mast of a ship, the local muscles provide stability and keep the mast from swaying. The global muscles are like the sails—they move the ship. If your global muscles are moving and your local muscles aren't, the mast just bends forward and back. You're not going anywhere.

If you've had a back injury or back pain, the deep local muscles that stabilize your back essentially shut off. It's your body's way of protecting them from further injury. The global muscles then have to compensate for this, but they're not endurance muscles like the local muscles. They're power sprinter muscles, so they can't provide stabilization and support for long. They'll eventually get tired and lose strength, and you'll get injured again.

You want to build core stiffness and stability so that you can efficiently transfer strength and speed to the limbs, increase the load-bearing capacity of the spine, strengthen the core muscles, and increase their endurance. All of that will ultimately reduce lower back pain and prevent leg and knee injuries.

Core stability training is crucial for getting your local muscles and global muscles working in balance again. It's important to work with an experienced chiropractor or trainer to pick the right exercises for you and learn to do them with correct form. The exercises I usually recommend include curl-ups, front plank, side plank, bird dogs (pointers), and my favorite, an exercise called stir the pot. I also like kettlebell swings to retrain the hip hinge. All these exercises focus on improving spinal stability and are spine-sparing—they won't hurt your back. They train the core as an integrated functional unit that can distribute and absorb and transfer forces.

If you'd like to learn more about these and other core stability exercises, check my website at drrobertsilverman. com, or these great sites: meyerdc.com and webexercises. com.

CASE STUDY: A MEDAL AT LAST

· · · · · ·

One of my patients is a fifty-five-year-old former Olympic athlete in weight lifting. Anthony is a big guy—six foot six— and very fit, but his body couldn't forget the injuries years of high-level competition had caused. He came to me because he was training to compete in a national Masters event for weight lifting. He really wanted a medal in the event, because in his entire athletic career, he never had. Despite his talent, he always came in fourth. As a former athlete myself, I understood how he felt. Anthony was having trouble with his form and wasn't sure why. I did a movement assessment, which makes the invisible visible to the trained eye. It was immediately clear that he had a tight right hip and a tight left shoulder, the legacy of years of repetitive trauma from training. We worked to retrain his brain and improve his form. He stopped compensating for old injuries and got into a better groove for his lifts. His hard work paid off when he finally won his championship six months later.

Let There Be Light

The leading edge in inside-out treatment today is low-level laser therapy, or LLLT. This therapy delivers excellent results and has tremendous potential for treating inflammation and helping patients with chronic pain from conditions such as knee arthritis.

Here's what happens when you have a soft-tissue injury, such as a sprain. The damaged cells release chemicals that initiate a natural inflammatory response in the body. As you know from Chapter 4, this leads to redness, swelling, warmth, and pain in the injured area. If the inflammation persists, joint damage can eventually happen. Therefore, we want to limit inflammation as much as we can. Low-level laser therapy helps by reducing the short-term inflammation, without drugs. I'll go into it in detail later in this chapter, but basically, laser therapy helps by stimulating the body's repair mechanisms. It treats the injury by activating biochemical energy and accelerating the healing process. The result is the resolution of inflammation and the development of normal, healthy tissue rather than scar tissue.

WHAT'S A LASER?

Laser is actually an acronym for Light Amplification by Stimulated Emission of Radiation. A laser beam is a focused beam of light that emits photon energy. The key to lasers as therapy is that the light beam can be tuned to specific wavelengths that have known health benefits but don't give off any heat that could damage tissue.

Lasers work on your body through basic photochemistry. The branch chain effect in photochemistry means that a single photon of light can trigger a reaction in a cell that causes the emission of several more photons. Those photons then trigger emissions in other cells in a chain reaction. The initial signal is multiplied and causes a rapid and regenerative flow of energy throughout the cells.

Imagine that, for some strange reason, I've set up 18,621 mousetraps on a football field; I've put a Ping-Pong ball in each mousetrap. The mousetraps are your cells. I toss one Ping-Pong ball onto the field and hit a mousetrap, which goes off and shoots its Ping-Pong ball onto another mousetrap. I've set off a cascade of bouncing balls. That's what happens when a laser hits a cell—the chain reaction moves through that cell and the ones around it, stimulating the healing process in several ways. First, the laser stimulates the release of nitric oxide in the cells, which expands blood vessels and lets more blood through. That helps bring nutrients to the area and carry away the waste products, especially the waste products produced by inflammation. For areas of the body that don't have good blood supply, like the discs in your vertebrae, increasing nitric oxide is very helpful. The laser also both increases cellular regeneration and increases cellular communication. Cellular regeneration occurs because the laser increases the production of adenosine triphosphate (ATP) in the mitochondria of the cell. Because ATP made in those little powerhouses transports chemical energy within your cells for metabolism, increasing production of it means increasing the cell's ability to heal and regenerate. Lasers increase cellular communication by improving the ability of your cells to "talk" to each other with chemical messengers. That helps the body coordinate its response to things like inflammation.

THE RIGHT WAVELENGTH

Lasers can produce very specific wavelengths of light. Some specific wavelengths are particularly helpful for healing. The 635 nm wavelength, for instance, is in the red part of the spectrum. It's been shown to be the most effective for photo biostimulation. It's the wavelength best for penetrating into the cells.

BENEFITS OF LASER THERAPY

Aside from how well it works, laser therapy has a lot of other benefits:

- Nontoxic
- Virtually no contraindications
- Noninvasive
- Easy to apply
- No side effects or pain
- Very safe
- Excellent alternative to pain killers and NSAIDs such as aspirin and ibuprofen

Lasers can also reduce the need for surgery for conditions like lower back pain and carpal tunnel syndrome.

Laser therapy speeds wound healing and reduces the formation of fibrous tissue when joint and soft-tissue injuries heal. They have anti-inflammatory action, increase vascular activity, and help regrow blood vessels, and they even help stimulate nerve function.

WHAT CONDITIONS ARE HELPED BY LASERS?

Any sort of joint or soft-tissue injury is usually helped by laser therapy. In my experience, it's valuable for the following conditions:

- Acute and chronic pain
- Back pain
- Achilles tendonitis
- Osteoarthritis and rheumatoid arthritis
- Bursitis
- Carpal tunnel syndrome
- Ligament sprains, especially sprained ankles
- Muscle strains
- Soft-tissue injuries
- Tendonitis
- Myofascial pain syndrome
- Tennis elbow/golfer's elbow
- Temporomandibular joint (TMJ) syndrome
- Rotator cuff injuries
- Knee pain
- Hip pain
- Plantar fasciitis and heel pain
- Concussion

Low-level laser therapy also helps heal peripheral nerves. It improves nerve cell metabolism, increases the sprouting of new connections between nerves, and actually enhances growth of new nerve axons and the myelin sheath that surrounds them. It can be very helpful for diabetic peripheral neuropathy. That's why I find it helpful for treating injuries that affect the nerves as well as the musculoskeletal system.

The FDA has already approved the use of low-level laser therapy for a dozen conditions, with more to come. One approved use is for treating neck pain caused by damage to the cervical spine (the vertebrae in your neck). In the case of cervical damage, the laser is approved to decrease pain and increase range of motion in the neck and shoulder region. Another approved use is treating plantar fasciitis, or heel pain.

The major study that showed that the laser treatment for plantar fasciitis is effective involved just two treatments a week for three weeks. The laser was applied to the top of the foot and two areas in the heel. Each treatment took just ten minutes. The results were literally off the charts. Patients reported much less heel pain on a standard measurement chart. Even more remarkable, the pain continued to decrease over the next six to twelve months. Later testing showed that the patients had improved blood circulation to the fascia in their feet.

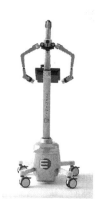

Laser therapy has been shown to help with hard-to-heal wounds, such as diabetic foot ulcers. Studies have also shown that it can be very beneficial for people with rheumatoid arthritis. LLLT reduces their constant pain and improves function. In fact, research shows that it works better than other nondrug modalities such as ultrasound, heat, exercise, acupuncture, and transcutaneous electrical nerve stimulation (TENS). Lasers are very helpful for treating tennis/golfer's elbow (lateral epicondylitis). In fact, LLLT for this condition is part of the British Medical Journal clinical evidence recommendations for treatment. The American Physical Therapy Association guidelines recommend LLLT for Achilles tendonitis. More and more, the research shows that laser therapy is a very valuable tool for treating pain, no matter what's causing it. Now that the dangers of powerful painkillers have become very obvious, I hope to see more use of lasers instead for pain management.

Several high-quality studies have shown that laser therapy can produce real relief from the pain of rheumatoid arthritis in the hands—treatment can reduce pain by as much as 70 percent. The studies for laser therapy and osteoarthritis are dramatic, many show that laser therapy can help with arthritic knees. One recent study looked at laser therapy for slowing down arthritis symptoms in a group of seventy elderly people with osteoarthritis in both knees. All the patients got standard physiotherapy. Each patient also received laser therapy to just one knee; the other knee got sham therapy. The study was blinded, so the patients didn't know which knee got the real laser and which got the sham. After five years, among the seventy knees that had received laser therapy, only one had been surgically replaced, while fifteen of the knees that received sham therapy had been replaced.

I use the Erchonia XLR8 laser to provide low-level laser therapy to my patients. It's a small, handheld device that's held just above the skin of the area to be treated. Most treatments take just a few minutes per area. Class II lasers like the XLR8 are so safe that the operator (me) doesn't even have to wear eye protection.

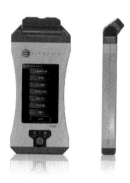

Founded in 1996, Erchonia (erchonia.com) is the first company in the world to gain FDA market clearance for the use of low-level laser therapy. To date, they've received fourteen FDA approvals, with more in progress. This company has done more level-one clinical trials with lasers than all the other manufacturers combined.

Three components of laser therapy are integral to a beneficial outcome from the treatment. The first component is the active ingredient: The specific wavelength is responsible for initiating biochemical cascades. Next comes the dose: The intensity (power of the light) determines the response. Too little light limits the response, but too much produces an adverse effect. By using a low-level laser, just the right amount of light is delivered. Finally comes the delivery mechanism: The way in which the light is delivered determines the tissue response and depth of penetration. The coherent, focused light of a laser ensures deep tissue stimulation.

The patient doesn't feel anything, because laser light at the wavelengths that are best for treatment don't produce any heat. The effects of low-level laser therapy are biochemical within the cells. The laser can't cause heating that would damage the skin or other living tissue. The type of energy delivered doesn't make the cells vibrate or oscillate, so it doesn't produce any sensation. The laser can penetrate through thin clothing, so the patients don't usually have to undress fully.

Dr. Mehmet Oz calls laser therapy the "no-pill pain buster." To me, the laser is the most versatile health-care modality of the twenty-first century. It's versatile in all the conditions it can treat, and versatile in the sense that the device is compact and lightweight. Unlike the older lasers, which were large, heavy machines, the Erchonia fits in my pocket. I can easily carry it from treatment room to treatment room. Because I now use laser as an adjunct to almost every treatment, this is very convenient. Today, I use laser treatment as a regular part of my treatment protocols. I have seen remarkable results.

CASE STUDY: PICK ME UP, MOMMY

• • • • • •

One of my patients is a young mother with a two-year-old. She was having a lot of trouble with her neck and right shoulder, to the point where she couldn't raise her arm up enough to pick up her kid. She couldn't even get a plate out of a kitchen cabinet. In addition to the usual treatments, I gave her three laser treatments in a week. Her pain just dissipated—within a week her full range of motion returned. She told me, "I can't remember the last time I got my arm up that high." Seeing the change in such a short period of time was very fulfilling. It was like turning on a light switch. Better yet, she was still pain-free six months later. The treatment worked so well because the 635 nanometer wavelength was able to reduce the inflammation quickly and reduce the imbalance in her joints. When we did that, the muscles that had been turned off came back on, and she was able to move correctly again. How did I know that LLLT would reduce her neck pain so quickly? I had read a study that appeared in the prestigious British medical journal *Lancet* back in 2009. Despite the article, mainstream medicine has been very slow to adopt laser therapy.

CASE STUDY: BACKING OUT OF THE DEAL

· · · · · ·

A lot of patients seek chiropractic treatments as a last resort. They've tried everything conventional medicine can offer and they're still in pain. That was why Ruth came to me. She's an athletic forty-four-year-old who hurt her back badly on a ski trip—not on the slopes, but she slipped on some ice walking back to the lodge. She ended up with three crushed disks and two vertebrae with compression fractures. Nothing helped with the pain. Rest, cortisone shots, heavy-duty painkillers, and even acupuncture left her in pain and barely able to move. Her doctor recommended surgery to fuse the damaged vertebrae. When she came to see me, the surgery was scheduled for just two weeks later. I didn't have much time for all my other functional treatments such as nutritional changes and supplements to help much, but we did have time for low-level laser therapy. We did three treatments over the course of the first week. After the third treatment she told me she felt 40 percent better, enough of an improvement in such a short time that she canceled the surgery. We then started a full rehab protocol, including laser treatment three times a week. Ruth is now pain free and back to her normal athletic self.

Inside-Out
Treatments

What seems to be a problem with one system can often be part of a problem with another. The problem needs to be traced as far upstream in the body's systems as possible. Once it's been pinpointed, then inside-out treatment will often be the most effective treatment. For example, recent research published in the prestigious journal *BMJ* showed that having high cholesterol is linked to a higher risk of tendon abnormalities and injuries and higher levels of pain associated with musculoskeletal problems in the arms. The reason may well be that cholesterol buildup in immune cells causes chronic low-level inflammation.

Now, when patients come to me with tendon problems, I check their cholesterol and inflammation numbers. If they're high, as they often are, I add nutritional modifications and supplements to my treatment arsenal to help lower cholesterol and calm inflammation.

The same thing holds true with leaky gut syndrome. As I've explained in Chapter 1, this problem isn't uncommon, given that most people eat the Standard American Diet. But leaky gut doesn't just cause inflammation, intestinal distress, and food intolerances. It also causes nutrient malabsorption. Your ability to absorb important nutrients, such as the B vitamins, iron, and magnesium, is compromised by leaky gut syndrome. So, even if you eat tons of foods that are high in B vitamins, you're still not going to absorb the nutrients well until you resolved the underlying issue. In an effort to get the nutrients it needs, your body makes you crave some food. I have to explain to my patients that the reason you keep eating, eating, eating is you're not absorbing anything. Leaky gut is complex and circular, but what it really comes down to is recognizing that leakiness causes downstream issues that are sometimes hard to trace further upstream. The tendency is just to treat the most apparent symptoms.

TREATING SOFT-TISSUE INJURIES

Soft-tissue injuries are one of my specialties. I work with many patients who have muscle, tendon, and ligament problems that show up as strains and sprains. These sorts of injuries are painful and can take a long time to heal if they're not treated properly. In the meantime, the patient becomes inactive, gains weight, loses fitness, and is generally unhappy. Unfortunately, what often happens is that the patient never really returns to full activity, never really loses the extra weight, and stays at a lower level of fitness. This is often because the patient fears reinjury, but it's also because the underlying issue that led to a tendency toward soft-tissue injury hasn't been discovered, much less treated. This is yet another situation where inside-out treatment can make a huge difference.

Injury Origins

Most soft-tissue injuries start with an imbalance in the muscles. When some muscles are hypertonic—too tight or too contracted—and others are weak, you get a postural imbalance. That leads to painful ligament sprains and muscle strains. Compensating for the injury by limping or otherwise favoring the painful area leads to more imbalance, which leads to slow healing of the original injury and increases the risk of reinjury or additional injury. When the weak muscles are in the lower back, it can eventually lead to the sort of degeneration in the joint that causes disc lesions or stenosis—in other words, a chronic bad back.

To fix soft-tissue injuries and help prevent reinjury and additional injury, I use what I call Dr. Rob's Super Five. These are five inside-out treatments that can really help your soft tissue structures heal and restore you to normal, pain-free activity: a daily multivitamin with minerals and phytonutrients, omega-3 fatty acids in the form of fish oil, vitamin D, probiotics, and a daily super green drink.

Joint Dysfunction

The first step in treating soft-tissue injury is analyzing joint dysfunction. The goal is to find the cause of the dysfunction. As I often say, "He who treats the site of pain is lost." Don't just treat the symptom. Find the cause. In my pretty extensive experience, it's not the muscles—it's the movement. Fixing how you move is the long-term goal. Musculoskeletal injuries take at least four to six weeks to heal. Unfortunately, after an injury, a tendon never really goes back to its original length. It will always be a bit shorter and tighter than it was. Your body keeps a perfect scorecard of every trauma it endures.

If you have a damaged structure such as a torn muscle or sprained ligament, my short-term goal for you is to get it to heal. That means a combination of manual rehabilitation techniques combined with nutritional changes and dietary supplements.

How Healing Happens

A soft-tissue injury has three phases:

- **Phase 1.** Phase 1 of the injury is the acute, or sudden onset, phase. This means the first seventy-two hours after the injury occurs. In the acute phase, inflammation is at its greatest. The injured area is swollen, red, painful, warm to the touch, and has restricted motion. Spasms may occur in surrounding tissues as the body tries to protect the injured area. The treatment goals at this point are to manage pain, minimize or reduce excessive swelling, relax tight muscles, and begin strategies to restore motion.

- **Phase 2.** Phase 2 of the injury is the healing period, which starts on day four and can last up to eight weeks. During this time, joint or muscle pain continues. The area around the injury may still be swollen, and range of motion may still be compromised. Tissue repair and remodeling has begun. The treatment goals at this point are to control pain and inflammation, improve joint stability, and use nutritional changes and supplements to aid in collagen synthesis and repair.

- **Phase 3.** Phase 3 of the injury focuses on wellness and ongoing care. The goals are to achieve optimal tissue remodeling by maintaining foundation nutrition and to reduce the risk of reinjury and degeneration.

As a rule of thumb, the earlier a musculoskeletal injury is treated, the sooner healing can begin. An untreated injury can easily slide from acute into subacute, and even into chronic.

During phase 1, nutrients that reduce swelling can be very helpful. The proteolytic enzymes (enzymes that break down proteins) bromelain, trypsin, and chymotrypsin can help reduce swelling, pain, and inflammation and may speed recovery. Turmeric or curcumin supplements help pain and inflammation by blocking enzymes such as cyclooxygenase and lipoxygenase, and they also stimulate the regeneration of muscle tissue. Ginger, *Boswellia serrata,* quercetin, and cayenne are all valuable for their anti-inflammatory effects. Calcium and magnesium supplements may help relieve spasms by promoting muscle relaxation. Lemon balm, passion flower, and valerian root are all herbs traditionally used to promote relaxation. They're considered safe and effective.

During phase 2, nutrients that support recovery and healing are valuable. When soft tissue is damaged, matrix metalloproteinase enzymes (MMPs) are naturally produced as part of the inflammatory process. If you have a poor diet and lifestyle, any injury or tissue damage can end up causing an overactivated release of MMPs. Continuing or excessive release of MMPs after the acute phase of the injury is over can slow healing and damage healthy collagen and connective tissue. We can reduce the production of MMPs during the healing phase with nutrients such as THIAA, berberine, selenium, zinc, biotin, and folic acid. During this time, nutrients that support collagen synthesis in the connective tissues and help with joint stability are invaluable. My patients usually benefit from supplements containing MSM and glucosamine with chondroitin.

During phase 3, the goal is to prevent reinjury and degeneration. That brings me back to Dr. Rob's Fab Five: a daily multivitamin with minerals and phytonutrients, omega-3 fatty acids in the form of fish oil, vitamin D, probiotics, and a daily super green drink, such as Nutri-Dyn Dynamic Fruits and Greens.

THE EXTRACELLULAR MATRIX

The extracellular matrix (ECM) is a general term for the connective tissue in the body: the tendons, ligaments, cartilage, and fascia. This is the network that binds our bodies together. The fascia provide adhesion to cells, act as a structural scaffold, and translate mechanical loading into cellular response.

The fascia also actively participate in intracellular signaling. The fascial system is the largest system in the body. It's the only system that touches every other system.

Normal muscle contraction depends on fascia, because 30 to 40 percent of the force generated by the muscle is actually due to the surrounding fascia. A muscle can stretch about 20 to 25 percent of its length. When it's stretched beyond that, it pulls on the bone, and the ligaments holding the joint together also get stretched and can get sprained. So, if you sprain your ankle, you've also strained your muscles beyond their maximum ability to stretch. A musculoskeletal injury will affect the fascia, which in turn will send signals that start the inflammatory cascade.

STRENGTHENING THE CORE

Your core refers to the muscles and fascia in your midriff, the part of your body between your chest and your waist. It's not just your abdominal muscles where the six-pack is. Your core is circular—it's all the muscles around your entire trunk, a sort of natural corset that's meant to hold your body in a stable position.

Your core is your body's anti-mover. It's your anti-rotation, anti-extension, anti-flexion system. Your core's first order of business is stability. Your core keeps you stable with two different types of muscles. The stability muscles hold you in position. The global muscles are more dynamic and let you have some mobility. Think of your core as the mast of a sailing ship. If your stability muscles are working properly, they hold the mast tightly in place. Your dynamic muscles act like sails attached to the mast—they can be moved around it to sail the ship. If the mast isn't held tightly upright by the stability muscles, then the sails of the dynamic muscles can't move correctly. If the muscles of your core are in balance, your core doesn't move much but remains flexible and doesn't break—it maintains stability.

The stability muscles are like endurance athletes. They

can hold up for long periods of time. The global muscles are like sprinters—they can move quickly, but then they shut off. If you have an episode of back pain, the stabilizing muscles deep in your core change how they function. Once they've been injured, they don't respond as quickly. Their action is delayed to the point where they only turn on after you move, which is too late. Studies suggest that this is particularly true of the contraction of the transversus abdominis muscle, a deep muscle in your abdomen that's your body's natural weight-lifting belt. When the contraction is delayed, that reduces spinal stability and increases the risk of more back pain. When the muscles are working only in short bursts, rather than being activated as you move, what happens then? Your brain says, "Ouch! These deep stabilizers don't seem to be functioning as well as they should. Let's get some of those global muscles to compensate." But those global muscles aren't good at endurance, so they don't provide a lot of stability. That's when you might turn up at my office, saying, "My back just gave way." What that really means is that your core muscles are shut off.

To fix your back in the long run, we have to retrain your core after a back injury.

Some 80 percent of all adults in their lifetime will have at least one episode of lower back pain. That's a very high percentage. Some of those people will go on to have back surgery in an attempt to get rid of the pain and restore normal motion. Those surgeries fail at least half of the time. I think that's a pretty unacceptable rate of failure. I'd much rather see my patients using natural methods to heal, and work on retraining their core, before they decide to do something that has a 50-50 chance of not helping.

EXERCISES FOR BACK PAIN

Strengthening your core is a great way to avoid back problems to begin with. If you've already had an episode (or two or three, as is often the case) of back pain, strengthening your core is crucial to avoiding another.

I recommend six core-strengthening exercises to my patients. They're so important that I have videos of how to do them on my website at drrobertsilverman.com.

The Brace

Bracing helps strengthen all the muscles in your abdomen and the deeper muscles in the lower back. To get an idea of how the muscles work here, place your thumbs in the small of your back on either side of your spine. Next, do a hip hinge: Bend forward from the hips about 15 degrees. You should feel the muscles in your lower back move as you bend. Stand back up again.

To do the brace, stand upright and suck in your stomach, as if you're about to get punched. Hold that for ten seconds, then relax. Repeat twenty times; do three sets.

You'll know you're doing the brace correctly if you poke

your extended fingertips right into your side below your ribs and then brace. You should feel the muscles move under your fingertips. If you do your braces faithfully every day, eventually you will unconsciously hold your body in that position, which will stabilize your lower back and help you prevent injury. You'll also be able to do all your normal activities of daily living, such as lifting grocery bags out of the car, easier.

DR. ROB ISM

No sit-ups, no crunches, for a healthy back.

Curl-Ups

Sit-ups and crunches used to be recommended for building the core muscles. No more. Now these exercises are seen as antiquated and outdated. We've learned that they put way too much flexion pressure on the vertebrae of the lower spine and actually lead to back injuries instead of preventing them. They also put a lot of stress on the neck vertebrae, leading to injuries there.

Instead of sit-ups and crunches, I recommend curl-ups. A curl-up looks sort of like a sit-up, but it engages all the core muscles and doesn't put strain on the lower back.

To do a curl-up, start by lying on your back. Place your hands palm-up beneath your lower back—you're doing this so you can feel the muscles there contract. Bend one leg and put the foot flat on the floor; extend the other leg. Hold your head and neck stiffly locked onto your ribcage—imagine them as one unit. Then lift your head and shoulders slightly off the floor by three or four inches and hold that position for twenty seconds. Your elbows should touch the floor while you do this. Relax and gently lie back again, then repeat ten times. Switch legs and repeat ten times gain. Do three sets.

Lift with your chest and abdomen muscles; don't flex your neck. In a curl-up, your rectus abdominis muscles (the long muscles that run vertically from your chest to your pubic area—the six-pack muscles) and your core muscles are the main activators. Unlike in a sit-up, you're not engaging your hip muscles.

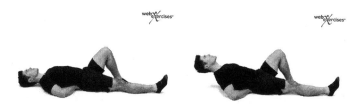

Front Plank

The front plank, also just called the plank, is a great exercise for the core. In this exercise, you're trying to imitate a plank of wood by holding your body stiff and flat. Start by getting into the push-up position, with your arms extended under your shoulders and your legs extended and your toes bent. Bend your arms ninety degrees, and rest your weight on your forearms. Brace in your core muscles, and contract your gluteus (butt) muscles. Your body should be perfectly straight from your shoulders to your ankles. I should be able to put a broomstick on your back, and it would just stay there instead of rolling off. As you'll soon feel, this exercise is also building arm and shoulder strength and working on your glutes as well.

Hold the plank position for as long as you can, aiming for at least thirty seconds. Over time, aim to hold your plank for ninety seconds.

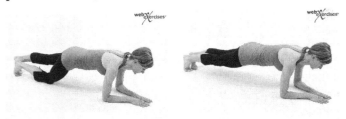

Side Plank

A side plank, also called a side bridge, is similar to a front plank, except you do it on your side. It's particularly good for strengthening the stabilizing muscles for the lower back. To do this exercise, start by lying on your right side with your feet staggered, so the top leg is in front of the bottom leg and the top leg's heel touches the bottom leg's toe. Lift your hips and support your body in a straight line with your right forearm. Your elbow should be directly under your shoulder. Hold for as long as you can, aiming for thirty seconds. Over time, aim to hold your side plank for seventy seconds. Switch sides and do it again.

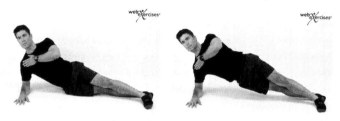

The Bird Dog or Pointer

Start this exercise on your hands and knees—the quadruped position. This exercise strengthens the back extensor muscles. Raise your right arm and point it forward, like a bird dog showing where the duck is. Simultaneously, raise your left leg and extend it backward. Support your weight on your left arm and right leg. Hold for eight seconds, then return to the quadruped position. Repeat eight times, then switch arms and legs and repeat for eight reps.

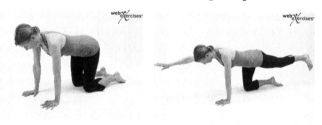

Stir the Pot

This is a great exercise for the core, but you need to have a physio exercise ball to do it. Get into the plank position with your elbows on the ball. Then move your body as if you're stirring a pot of oatmeal, first for ten seconds clockwise and then for ten seconds counterclockwise. Repeat for ten reps.

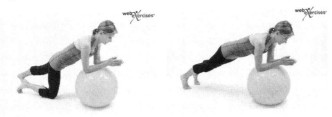

PROPRIOCEPTION

Proprioception is your unconscious sense of where your body is in space. Proprioception affects your sense of balance, spatial orientation, and how you move. It's the balance between your nervous system and your musculoskeletal system. Muscle, tendons, and ligaments all send messages to the brain, telling the brain how to react to a stimuli.

After an injury, proprioception is always altered. The right muscles aren't doing the right thing at the right time. It's like looking at your computer screen. You hit the keyboard to take you to one website but miss a letter and end up somewhere else. The input isn't matching the output. This is why if you've had one injury, such as a sprained ankle, you're likely to injure the same place again. Your sense of where it is and how it responds isn't the same anymore.

We can do a lot to help you regain proprioception and

avoid reinjury. I like my patients to work with wobble boards or rocker boards. These are platforms large enough to stand on with both feet that have half a sphere attached to the bottom. The sphere makes the platform a bit like a teeter-totter. You have to continuously adjust your balance to stabilize yourself on the board. The boards help you reset the altered motor control from the injury. The boards help retrain injured muscles, tendons, and ligaments to react to instability. Proprioception training has also been shown to improve posture and reduce the incidence of overuse injuries.

DR. ROBISM

Practice the way you play. Work with your chiropractor or trainer to choose exercises that reflect your everyday activities.

TENDINOPATHY

When a tendon, the tough connective tissue that holds muscle to bone, gets overloaded, it can get damaged and even torn. Imagine two people pulling on opposite ends of a rope. The rope fibers fray and pull apart. That's a lot like what happens to a damaged tendon. The body has a hard time repairing damaged tendons because the collagen fibers are disrupted. The repair tends to be disorganized, leaving the tendon shortened, distorted, and less effective.

I believe that restoring optimum function is a major component of eliminating pain and preventing injury.

CHIROPRACTIC TREATMENTS

Joint Manipulation

When people think of chiropractic treatment, they're usually thinking of joint manipulation. This treatment is done by passive movement of a skeletal joint. The manipulation is intended to improve the function of a joint by releasing restricted joint movement and improving biomechanical and neurological function. Manipulation restores normal motion to the joints of the spine, arms, and legs. It relaxes tight muscles, improves coordination, and inhibits pain.

During joint manipulation, an audible clicking or popping sound is usually heard. The sounds are believed to be the result of a phenomenon known as cavitation occurring within the synovial fluid (the lubricating liquid found inside joints) of the joint. During the manipulation, the pressure within the joint cavity is reduced. In a low-pressure environment, some of the gases that are naturally dissolved in the synovial fluid come out and form bubbles that then rapidly collapse, causing the popping sound.

Active Release Technique®

The Active Release Technique (ART) is a manual technique used by chiropractors. It's a highly successful approach to the diagnosis and treatment of muscles, tendons, ligaments, nerves, and fascia. A skilled practitioner with a thorough knowledge of anatomy uses symptom patterns and functional testing to locate scar tissue and adhesions from old injuries in between muscles and nerves. The practitioner touches the problem area while the patient moves that part of the body through a specific range of motion. The movement helps break up adhesions, especially at the fascial level. It's great for relieving muscle discomfort and really outstanding for relieving nerve entrapment.

Graston Technique®

The Graston Technique is another approach to treating scar tissue and adhesions. It's an instrument-assisted form of soft tissue mobilization. It's excellent for treating soft tissue fibrosis or chronic inflammation and restoring range of motion. The instrument for the Graston Technique is a blunt stainless steel probe that glides along muscles, tendons, and ligaments and acts like a scar tissue "stethoscope." When the practitioner feels knots or bands of scar tissue, the instrument can then be used to break up the restriction or adhesion. Stretching exercises are then used to promote realignment of the fibers so that they behave more like normal, healthy tissue.

The benefit of the Graston Technique is not only in the fact that it accurately detects restriction and adhesions, but also in the amount of improvement that takes place in a short amount of time. When the Graston Technique is coupled with the necessary strengthening and stretching exercises, the patient gets better much more quickly and completely. Most patients see excellent results in six to eight treatments.

The FAKTR technique, which stands for functional and kinetic treatment with rehabilitation, is another instrument-based technique that works along the same lines as the Graston Technique. It uses metal instruments that are shaped to sense areas of restriction and press down on them very accurately. By putting varying degrees of pressure on the area with the instrument as the patient moves against it, we can break up underlying scar tissue. FAKTR treatment looks at the patient's whole chain of motion, not just the site of the pain.

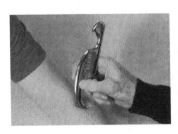 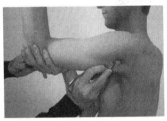

DR. ROB'SM

Assess, treat, and reassess. Then do it again.

I work with a lot of very talented athletes to help them stay healthy and build their skills. What I've learned from working with athletes applies to my nonathlete patients as well—including the ones who are the opposite of athletic. One of the things I do with all my patients is functional movement assessment. (There's a video showing how this works on my website at drrobertsilverman.com/video. htm.)

Life is motion—and if you can't move well, you can't live well. Functional movement assessment allows me to test your movement and see where you're out of balance in ways that can cause pain, nerve entrapment, reinjury, and other problems. When I assess your movement, it makes the invisible visible.

DR. ROB'SM

Movement never lies. It tells the unique story of each individual's history, compensations, and adaptations.

I use the results of the assessment to help you attain mobile ankles, mobile hips, a stable core, and mobile shoulders. We do it through appropriate corrective treatment, exercise, and motor control protocols, mixed with nutrition and laser therapy (as explained in earlier chapters).

Functional movement assessment uses standard orthopedic and neurological tests to get to structural damage and aberrant movement patterns. During the testing I look for typical dysfunctions, including thoracic collapse, the inability to perform a hip hinge, spine twisting and rotation, and loss of neutral spine position (typically rounding the back).

As discussed in more detail in Chapter 6, I look at seven movement areas to assess you:

- Posture. Can you stand up straight without pain?
- Overhead squat. Your ability to lift a weight over your head while squatting is a good measure of your core strength and shoulder mobility.
- One-legged squat. Your ability to do a squat on one leg is a good measure of your core strength, leg strength, ankle and knee integrity, and proprioception.
- Trunk stability push-up. This is a much harder version of a push-up. It's done to assess the stability of your trunk—the central part of your body.
- Valgus jump test. *Valgus* means a deformity away or out from the midline. A valgus jump test is a good way to see if your knee is out of alignment.

- Upper and lower muscle firing patterns.
- Regular push-up. Your ability to do push-ups is a good measure of your upper body strength.

Nerves glide through your muscles. If you think of muscle as the prongs of a fork, the nerves are spaghetti. If the muscles are too tight, they grab on to the spaghetti and squeeze it. That entraps the nerve—the nerve can't move freely because it's stuck somewhere along its path. This can cause pain or change in sensation, but it can also cause more subtle problems of decreased range of motion and decreased strength. Nerve entrapment usually shows up as sciatica, carpal tunnel syndrome, a pinched nerve in the neck, or back pain from a bulging or herniated disc.

We can use neurodynamic testing to assess the mobility of the nerves as they wind through the muscles. I use it to diagnose restrictions and resistances that inhibit the glide of the nerve. To make the nerve move smoothly again, I'll teach you how to do nerve flossing. It's sort of like flossing your teeth. Just as you floss your teeth by pulling on one end of the dental floss and releasing the other, and then repeating, this exercise will pull on an affected nerve to free it from entrapment and adhesion. The goal is to pull one end of the nerve while relaxing the other end of the nerve. For sciatic nerve pain, you would imagine a string running from your big toe to your forehead. To pull on the nerve and move it through the muscle, sit in a chair and flex your neck forward. That creates a pull on the spinal cord starting at the base of your skull and a release on the spinal cord ending at the base of your spine. Gently bring your head back up while simultaneously extending your legs from the knee. This pulls the nerve from the base of your spine and releases it at the base of your skull. Repeat five times. You can see a video showing how to do this flossing exercise and others on my website drrobertsilverman.com.

Resistance Bands

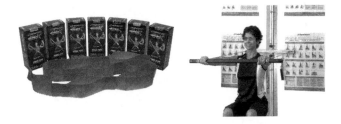

Stretchy resistance bands—often called Therabands (thera-band.com) after the leading manufacturer—are very widely used in rehab. I use them every day with virtually every patient, ranging from the most developed, muscular athletes to my mother, who is eighty-seven. Bands are great because they come in all levels of resistance, from low to high. For rehab, they're better than free weights because you can choose the level of resistance that's right for each person. That proprioceptive feedback is very helpful. I use bands a lot, from the little bands that just go around your ankles and your feet to bigger ones for upper body work. I ultimately like to help my patients outgrow the bands and move on to free weights or kettlebells.

Kinesio Taping

Kinesio taping is a therapeutic rehab technique invented by Dr. Kenzo Kase nearly thirty years ago in Japan. This method uses a special athletic tape for treating muscular disorders. The tape is placed over and around the affected muscles to support them and prevent overcontraction while still maintaining a full range of motion. This is very helpful for letting people continue their normal activities while they heal.

For acute injuries, Kinesio taping helps prevent overuse and overcontraction during the early, most painful stage of an injury. The taping also helps improve blood flow and move lymph through the area to carry away the waste products of inflammation. The outside assistance from the tape helps the muscles activate the body's own healing processes. The tape is safe and comfortable. Once it's in place, it can be worn for several days at a time.

I've seen tremendous benefits from Kinesio taping in many of my patients. It's not a primary treatment for an acute injury or even during recovery, but it does seem to help relieve pain and reduce swelling. I see it as the icing on the cake after all the other treatments.

Flexion-Distraction

Another way to describe the flexion-distraction technique is to call it back decompression. For many of my patients, flexion-distraction is a safe and effective alternative to elective back surgery. Flexion-distraction can also be used to treat people with a variety of pain syndromes that have not responded to other treatment approaches. It's a gentle chiropractic treatment procedure for spinal pain, back and neck pain, and arm and leg pain.

The flexion-distraction adjustment is done on a special table that was designed by James M. Cox, DC, DACBR, a leader in the field. It's based on the idea that an external distractive or decompressing force can help separate the spine and allow the discs and other connective tissues to move off impinged nerves. This can significantly reduce or even eliminate pain. The flexion-distraction technique uses the Cox table to restore normal physiological range of motion to the cervical, thoracic, and lumbar spinal joints. It's a gentle, nonforce adjusting procedure that works with the body's natural design. I use this technique to help with pain and other symptoms caused by herniated and bulging discs, sciatica, stenosis, and osteoarthritis of the vertebrae.

CASE STUDY: GETTING BACK TO HEALTH

· · · · · ·

When Andy came to see me, he was close to despair. At twenty-six, he was a serious CrossFit competitor who had quit investment banking to open his own CrossFit box. His career was starting to take off when he herniated six disks in his back. How? Even serious CrossFit types can have bad lifting technique.

His orthopedic doctor said no more weight lifting. But weights are central to the CrossFit program, and without being able to lift, Andy would be out of competition and out of business. Andy had read about Active Release Technique in Timothy Ferris's book *The 4-Hour Body*. He was eager to try it. As an expert in this protocol, I was able to assess Andy and decide that ART was a good treatment option for him. Six weeks later, he was back in competition at the elite level, better than before. It wasn't just the ART. We also used other inside-out treatments, including Kinesio taping, core exercises, and nutritional improvements. We also worked on his proprioception to improve his lifting form so he could avoid getting injured again. Five years later, Andy hasn't had another injury, he's won several competitions, and he now has several successful CrossFit boxes.

Concussion from
the Inside-Out

Injury to brain means injury to gut. Fix them both.

In recent years, I've seen a big increase in the number of patients who come to me for treatment of concussion. In part, that's because more women are playing sports like soccer, which has a high concussion rate. A bigger part is that concussion has been in the news a lot. Recent revelations about the long-term brain effects of repeated concussions on professional football players have made everyone more aware of the problem.

Every year about 250,000 kids are treated for concussion in emergency rooms, usually from playing sports;

probably twice that number or more are treated by their pediatricians. The total number of concussions reported every year is around 3.8 million, but this number is probably too low. Many concussions in sports and in life simply go undiagnosed and untreated. A lot of my patients come to me because they've finally been diagnosed and now need help with managing long-term symptoms.

WHAT'S A CONCUSSION?

A concussion is the most minor form of a traumatic brain injury. It means you have a temporary loss of normal brain function. Most concussions are caused by a big bump or blow to the head, as in a car accident where your head hits something in the vehicle, or a soccer collision where your head hits the ground. A hit to the body that jolts the head, like a football tackle, can also cause a concussion. The sudden impact of the blow or jolt makes the brain bounce around in the skull, which damages neurons, causes an alteration in mental status, and releases natural chemicals that affect the brain and the rest of the body.

Only about one in ten people who get a concussion lose consciousness. The damage from a concussion is internal—you don't always get a visible bump, bruise, or cut where you hit your head. Concussions also don't show up on imaging such as X-rays, CT scans, and MRIs. Blood tests for concussion are in development, but for now, most concussions are diagnosed by their symptoms.

Because there aren't any visible signs of concussion, many people get mild concussions and don't realize it. They don't seek treatment, which can make recovery take longer and could lead to chronic symptoms and even serious complications. Having one concussion makes you much more likely to get a second one, especially if you return to sports too quickly. Having a concussion also makes you more likely to get a leg injury when you go back to playing. Again, if the first concussion isn't diagnosed, the chances of later injury rise sharply. The most serious consequence of an undiagnosed concussion is second impact syndrome—getting a second concussion before the symptoms of the first have resolved. The impact to the brain can cause rapid and fatal brain swelling.

CONCUSSION SYMPTOMS

If you have a concussion, you could have one or more of a range of symptoms. Right after the impact to the head, the most common symptoms are the following:

- Inability to think straight—the injured person feels foggy, dazed, disoriented
- Inability to follow directions
- Disturbance of awareness and inability to focus
- Nausea and vomiting

BLOOD TESTS FOR CONCUSSION

· · · · · ·

Looking to the future, I see a much bigger role for blood tests that can detect proteins caused by head trauma. Right now, two different tests are available. One looks at a protein called UCH-L1. Levels of this protein rise quickly after a concussion but decline substantially within two days. Elevated levels of another protein, GFAP, are detectable for about a week following injury. Concussion isn't always easy to diagnose by symptoms alone, and sometimes symptoms are delayed by a couple of days, so these tests can be helpful. Going forward, I think the research in this area will lead to even more sensitive tests for these proteins and others. We'll be able to diagnose concussion in cases where the patient ignores the symptoms at first and only seeks treatment days or even weeks after the trauma happened. The blood tests will also be helpful for showing patients who are in denial about having a concussion—when they see the results, they'll finally understand why they're feeling the way they do. What I find most exciting about the future of blood testing for concussion is that we'll be able to use the tests to track recovery and diagnose post-concussion syndrome. Right now, we tell patients to gradually return to normal activity based on how they feel, but often they feel better than they really are. They go back to work or sports too soon and start having symptoms again. Athletes who go back to playing too soon are at risk of second impact syndrome. With blood tests, we'll be able to say whether it's safe to get back on the field. Blood tests could also be very helpful for managing post-concussion syndrome, where recovery is substantially delayed. The testing could help us figure out what part of the delay is from the brain damage and what part is from other damage, such as injury to the head and neck muscles.

Other symptoms, such as headache, double vision, dizziness, balance problems, sensitivity to light or noise, constant tiredness, sleep disturbances, lack of concentration, depression, and irritability may appear soon after, usually within the next couple of days. After the initial impact symptoms, dizziness is probably the most common concussion symptom.

In the long run, concussion can have a very dangerous side effect: an increased risk of suicide. Even a single mild concussion could triple the lifetime risk.

GRADING CONCUSSION

Concussions are graded into three categories:

- A grade 1 concussion is mild; there's no loss of consciousness and the symptoms last for under fifteen minutes.
- A grade 2 concussion is moderate; there's no loss of consciousness but the symptoms last longer than fifteen minutes.
- A grade 3 concussion is severe; there's brief loss of consciousness.

With proper treatment, most people with mild concussion get over it in about one to two weeks. Recovery from more severe concussions can take longer. Severe concussion also has a greater chance of complications, such as post-concussion syndrome, where symptoms such as headaches and dizziness begin a few days after the concussion and may continue for many weeks or even months.

WOMEN AND CONCUSSION

Women have a higher rate of concussions. In fact, women playing high school sports experience concussions at twice the rate of their male counterparts. Their risk of a concussion from soccer, for instance, is more than twice that for male soccer players. The reason is that the neck muscles in a woman are less developed than those in a man and provide less protection to the head from sudden movement. In addition, a woman's head is usually lighter and smaller. Both factors combine to cause a stronger whiplike action when women are tackled or hit the ground. Women also tend to report injuries at a higher rate.

The female menstrual cycle may impact the severity of concussion symptoms. Women injured during the pre-menstrual stage (when progesterone levels are naturally high) experienced slower recovery and poorer health one month after injury as compared to women injured during the two weeks directly after their period. An abrupt drop in progesterone after an injury may lead to worsening post-concussion symptoms such as headache, nausea, dizziness, and trouble concentrating.

Women also tend to recover from concussion more

slowly. In particular, they tend to be slower to regain memory function.

WHY MORE CONCUSSIONS?

As I mentioned earlier, there has been an increase in the number of people being treated for concussions. One possible reason for the increase in the number of concussions in general goes beyond the fact that more women are playing concussion-prone sports in addition to the men who already play these sports. It's possible that a condition called diminished brain resilience syndrome (DBRS) is playing a role. DBRS is a modern-day neurological pathology of increased susceptibility to mild brain trauma, concussion, and downstream neurodegeneration.

Our modern environment exposes us to a lot of toxins. Most Americans also eat a diet full of heavily processed, nutrient-deficient foods with a bad balance of dietary fats. And most Americans are sedentary and unfit. Combine that with imbalanced gut bacteria and poor liver function, and you're set up for reduced protection from impact damage. In other words, what might just be a minor bump to the head turns into a concussion. And because your body is already out of balance, recovering from that concussion could take longer.

Another possible reason for more concussions is poorly fitting protective headgear. Football helmets often don't fit correctly for maximum protection. Football helmets with air bladder linings don't seem to protect against concussion.

A BANG ON THE BRAIN

Your brain weighs only about three pounds, but it has 100,000 miles of blood vessels. It contains about 100 billion neurons, or more neurons than there are stars in the Milky Way. The soft tissue of your brain floats within your skull in a bath of cushioning cerebrospinal fluid. But when your head whips back and forth, your brain sloshes around. It hits the skull, then bounces back and hits the skull again. When you have a concussion from a hard impact to the head, in effect you get a bruise on your brain. The neurons get stretched out and can't communicate well with each other. In response to the injury, your brain releases a lot of inflammatory chemicals that cause swelling. Your head and neck muscles may also be sore and swollen. (If the rectus capitis posterior minor muscle—the muscle at the back of the head that lets you rock and tilt your head—is affected, concussion symptoms tend to be more severe and have worse outcomes.)

We've come to realize that the impact of a concussion on the brain sets off a cascade of consequences elsewhere in the body. In particular, having a concussion almost immediately (within six hours) causes leaky gut syndrome (check back to Chapter 1 for a discussion of this). The reason seems to be that concussion disrupts the signals that the vagus nerve, which links the brain to the gut, sends between the two. The damage opens the blood-brain barrier, a network of blood vessels that lets essential nutrients into the brain while keeping out most other substances—and vice versa. Peptides (short protein molecules) produced in the brain in response to the concussion end up in the gut. This causes a decrease in the expression of the gut proteins zonulin and occludin. These proteins are responsible for keeping the spaces between the cells in the intestinal wall nice and tight. When the proteins decrease, those tight junctions relax a bit, causing leaky gut syndrome within hours of the head injury. So, a leaky brain leads to a leaky gut. As the concussion heals, other symptoms like headaches get better, but once a gut gets leaky, it typically doesn't heal on its own. To treat this and avoid long-term damage, I recommend immediately following the leaky gut protocol I described in Chapter 1.

NUTRITIONAL PROTOCOL FOR TREATING CONCUSSION

When the brain is injured, it responds by releasing a lot of natural chemicals to repair the injured neurons. In particular, it releases brain-derived neurotrophic factor (BDNF), which helps neurons grow, restores communication among them, and reduces the risk of neurodegeneration. The thalamus in the brain also releases substance P, the neurotransmitter that makes us feel pain. When you get a concussion, your damaged neurons make you release a lot of substance P, which not only increases your sensitivity to pain but also causes some swelling. Substance P is also tied to the body's response to nausea, which is probably a big reason for the nausea and vomiting that often go with a concussion. Lowering the level of substance P decreases the inflammation in the brain and cuts back on nausea and pain.

Once a concussion is diagnosed, I strongly recommend taking immediate nutritional steps to help speed the recovery. Nutritional supplements can really help reduce inflammation and the release of substance P, support the production of BDNF, and treat leaky gut before it becomes a bigger problem.

After a head injury, your body needs extra protein right away for healing and rebuilding damaged tissues. Starting within a day of the injury, I recommend consuming extra protein each day at the rate of about a gram per kilogram of body weight. You can eat high-protein foods such as steak and eggs, but the nausea that often goes along with a concussion may keep you from getting that down. I recommend a daily shake made with whey protein or pea and rice protein with added branched chain amino acids, combined with ten grams of the supplement creatine monohydrate. I like adding creatine because it's crucial for energy production within the cells. It helps give the brain an intense and immediate hit of energy, which it needs to help the cells start to heal.

To reduce inflammatory damage to the brain, I recommend supplements of natural anti-inflammatories such as quercetin, boswellia, ginger, grape seed extract, bromelain, turmeric, and resveratrol.

Inflammation produces a lot of free radicals, so taking antioxidants to help limit the damage they cause can be helpful. An excellent antioxidant for concussion is alpha lipoic acid (ALA). It works well in both the watery parts of cells and also the fatty parts. Your brain is about one-third fat, so ALA is very effective in brain cells. I recommend 600 mg daily. I also recommend 500 to 1,000 mg daily of vitamin C, which is a crucial antioxidant in the body.

The supplement choline, a member of the B vitamins family, is critical for brain development in the womb. In concussion treatment, it may improve cognitive function. I suggest choline supplements; 25 mg daily can be helpful. Vitamin D is neuroprotective; I suggest a daily supplement of 5,000 IU. Zinc and magnesium are both really important for making the enzymes needed for central nervous system neurotransmitters. Most Americans are deficient in vitamin D, zinc, and magnesium, another overall reason today why people are more susceptible to concussion. Magnesium is one the best weapons against delayed brain injury and post-concussion syndrome. It reduces inflammation and raises glutathione (your body's most important antioxidant) in cells. Low levels of magnesium in the brain have been shown to greatly increase the vulnerability of the brain to injury. I recommend daily supplements containing up to 600 mg of magnesium and 40 mg of zinc.

I also recommend the omega-3 fatty acids EPA and DHA, found in fish oil, for reducing inflammation. The DHA in fish oil helps build strong, flexible cell membranes in neurons. The EPA suppresses the production of inflammatory prostaglandins and other inflammatory chemicals. During the first few weeks of the concussion recovery period, I suggest supplements of a high-quality fish oil up to 4,000 mg daily. After that, continue with 2,000 to 4,000 mg a day for three months.

Interestingly, there's some evidence that taking DHA supplements regularly can help prevent concussion by making the brain more resilient against a hit. Also, when you take fish oil and vitamin D together, they have a synergistic effect on your production of the neurotransmitter serotonin, which is associated with depression. Producing more could help prevent the depression that's a common symptom of concussion. The omega-3 fatty acids are also helpful for increasing the production of BDNF.

Studies have recently shown that administering glutathione after a concussion reduces brain tissue damage by an average of 70 percent. In a clinical setting, glutathione can be given intravenously. Oral supplements of glutathione are destroyed by stomach acid, however. For home treatment, we can't give this as a supplement. Instead, we can nutritionally support the body's natural pathway for producing glutathione with the building blocks: vitamin C, selenium, niacinamide (vitamin B3), N-acetyl-L-cysteine (750 to 1,000 mg), and broccoli extract.

We know from many solid studies that speedy intake of macro- and micronutrients is crucial. Start taking them as soon as possible after the concussion and continue them daily for two weeks. If concussion symptoms persist past a reasonable amount of healing time (more than two weeks for a minor concussion), it's possible that the thalamus of the brain is struggling. This means the ratio of substance P to BDNF is excessive. To decrease the production of substance P, continue taking DHA, bromelain, quercetin, ginger, vitamin D, alpha lipoic acid, and magnesium. To build up BDNF, continue taking zinc, turmeric, and resveratrol. I also suggest adding supplements of the amino acid L-carnitine, because it helps with repairing and growing neurons.

Laser Therapy for Concussion

I've found that adding low-level laser therapy to my basic concussion protocol really helps my patients recover faster. As I explained in Chapter 7, laser light has been shown to suppress pro-inflammatory cytokines such as interleukin-1 and interleukin-6. Low-level laser therapy also up-regulates BDNF, which helps nerves grow, makes the synapses between nerves work well, reduces the risk of neurodegeneration, and supports the branching network of neurons. After a traumatic brain injury or concussion, BDNF production decreases, but that's when you need it most. The laser also helps prevent atrophy in the dendrites, the tiny branching projections that connect the synapses between neurons.

A 2007 study of concussion patients and laser therapy in Israel showed that patients who got laser treatment soon after the impact had far fewer neurological deficits five days later. Thirty days later, they were doing significantly better than the control group that didn't get laser therapy. Numerous studies before and since this one have shown that transcranial laser therapy is effective.

I usually see patients with mild brain injuries three times a week for three weeks for laser treatments. I apply the laser for thirty seconds to each major area of the brain—the cerebrum, the temporal lobe, the occipital lobe, the frontal and parietal lobes, and the cerebellum. I also laser the muscles of the occipital region where the spinal column meets the skull, the back of the neck, and the muscles of the upper chest area for about a minute each. The whole treatment takes about ten minutes. LLLT really seems to help them get over the worst of a concussion faster.

Recently, we've had a major breakthrough in laser therapy for concussion: vagus nerve stimulation. Some important research has shown that stimulating the vagus nerve, which links the brain and the gut, reduces inflammation and protects against intestinal epithelial barrier breakdown. In other words, by stimulating the vagus nerve in the appropriate locations with a laser as soon as possible after a concussion, we can help prevent leaky gut syndrome from getting started.

The laser wavelength needed to reach the vagus nerve is violet light at 405 nanometers (the standard laser uses light at 635 nm). I feel this new treatment is so important that I've invested in the specialized laser needed to perform it. My results so far with competitive athletes have been excellent.

Rest and Exercise

The primary treatment for concussion in the first few days is rest. Recent research suggests, however, that complete rest until the patient is symptom-free after a concussion may not be best for recovery. Exercising carefully within a week of injury, regardless of symptoms, seems to nearly halve the rate of concussion symptoms that linger more than a month.

I recommend a gradual return to exercise and normal activity, starting as soon as possible. At all times, of course, the patient's symptoms should guide the activity level. As soon as the patient feels up to it, light aerobic activity such as walking or riding an exercise bike can be started. I usually suggest doing this just for a brief period, no more than ten minutes the first day, and slowly increasing. At this stage, weight lifting, running, jumping, and similar activities—anything that would jar the head—are absolutely forbidden. As symptoms permit, gradually work up day by day to moderate activity, such as jogging. A full return to active sports should be gradual and happen only when concussion symptoms are gone. If they return, the activity needs to be stopped, and the person needs to rest for at least twenty-four hours.

CONCUSSION REHAB

With proper treatment, most people with a mild concussion recover fully within a couple of weeks and can return to their normal activities. More serious concussions take longer—sometimes much longer—to improve. Rest, gentle exercise, and nutritional supplements are very important for long-term recovery. In addition, we can use some excellent neurosensory rehab approaches to help improve lingering concussion symptoms, such as dizziness and vision problems. We usually get good results from three sessions a week for four to eight weeks in addition to other treatments, such as laser therapy. I have a good success rate with athletes—90 percent get back into the game safely. But you don't have to be an athlete to benefit from rehab. Anyone with a concussion, at any age, can be helped.

I take a multisystem approach to concussion rehab. I

look at the musculoskeletal system, balance, visual disturbances, and dizziness to decide which areas are affected and need to be treated.

Musculoskeletal System

Most people who get a big bang on the head also got banged in the muscles of the head, neck, and shoulders; their spines were usually banged as well. Patients often tell me they feel achiness and pressure in the occipital muscles at the base of the skull. They often have pain and limited range of motion in the neck muscles. Once I've ruled out injuries such as a fractured or damaged vertebrae in the neck, I can use standard manual techniques to relax tight muscles and reduce inflammation (check back to Chapter 8 for more on ART and other methods).

Balance

Concussion disrupts the brain's ability to interpret and integrate incoming and outgoing information from the nerves in the body. That can lead to trouble with balance—a patient might not be able to stand on one leg, for instance, or balance with the eyes closed, or might just feel wobbly and unable to stand upright for long. We can help this by teaching the patient to rely less on vision for balance and more on other cues, such as touch and vibration, to be aware of where their body is. I work with the patient on balance exercises done with the eyes closed or in a dark room. We can also use the wobble board to work on improving balance.

Persistent dizziness after a concussion may be coming not from the brain but from damage to the vertebrae in the neck (cervicogenic dizziness). The nerves there are garbling the proprioceptive signals they send to the muscles. We can do some simple testing to see if that's the case. This usually responds well to balance training and proprioceptive rehab.

Visual Disturbances

After a concussion, patients often have trouble tracking things with their eyes. They may also have blurry vision, double vision, or other visual disturbances. The problem isn't in the eyes themselves; it's in the brain's ability to control eye alignment, movement, focus, and visual processing. This is almost always because the concussion has damaged one or more of the three cranial nerves that control the movement of the eyes. Patients who have visual disturbances need to be diagnosed by an eye doctor. Once we know what the problems are, we work with training software to do vision exercises. The programs are a lot like video games—they help the patient with tracking, focusing, and eye teaming to reduce double vision. My patients usually do really well with this. Their visual disturbances usually get better in five to ten visits.

Vestibular Disturbances

Vestibular means relating to the inner ear, or more generally, relating to balance and dizziness. Feeling dizzy in the first few days is one of the most common concussion symptoms—up to 80 percent of all patients are dizzy to some degree. Because dizziness can cause nausea and vomiting and really restrict activity, and because it can cause falls, vestibular disturbance is a top priority in concussion rehab. Interestingly, dizziness is a predictor of the speed of recovery. If dizziness is the main symptom when an athlete gets injured on the field, his or her recovery is likely to take three weeks or longer.

I use a protocol called the vestibular oculomotor screen (VOMS, appropriately) to assess dizziness and track progress. Our goals with therapy are to improve dizziness and disequilibrium symptoms and desensitize the patient to things that make dizziness worse, such as being in a busy environment.

Gaze stabilization exercises help quite a bit. I have the patient look fixedly at a target at eye level while turning the head 45 degrees to the left and then right. Doing this at home twice a day for ten to twenty times really helps relieve dizziness. To help overcome dizziness from too much sensory input at once, gradually increasing exposure over a few weeks helps.

POST-CONCUSSION SYNDROME

Anywhere from 10 to 20 percent of patients with a concussion develop post-concussion syndrome. Although there's no clear-cut definition for this, it usually means that full recovery from concussion symptoms just isn't happening. The deficits persist beyond the normal time frame for recovery (up to three months) and become chronic. As many as 225,000 new patients every year show long-term deficits as a result of concussion. One of the most common long-term effects is dizziness, which can sometimes persist for years after the concussion.

The symptoms of post-concussion syndrome are complex and vary quite a bit among patients. They include the following:

- Impaired attention, memory, and executive function
- Feeling foggy, unable to focus
- Blurred vision
- Depression
- Poor sleep
- Dizziness
- Chronic pain (headache)
- Feeling frustrated or impatient, panic attacks
- Irritability, easily angered
- Sensitivity to noise and light
- Decreased alcohol tolerance

Many patients with post-concussion syndrome have it because they were never diagnosed with a concussion to begin with, or they were inadequately treated. Post-concussion syndrome is usually diagnosed by a physician, but it takes a team to help the patient. That's when the patient often gets sent to me for therapy.

CASE STUDY: BACK ON THE
FIELD IN THREE WEEKS

• • • • • •

One of my favorite patients is a Division 1 soccer player at an elite university. She's the team captain—she's a great athlete and a great person, with an amazing future ahead of her. As a high school athlete who played several sports, she had already had five concussions by the time she got to college; each one ended her play for the season. She got another mild concussion in her first year of college and was out for the rest of the season. In her sophomore year, she dove for a ball and took a knee right in the middle of her forehead so hard she was briefly knocked out. When she came to, she had typical symptoms of acute grade 3 concussion: she was dazed, didn't know where she was, couldn't count backward from ten, was sensitive to light, and was throwing up. The next day, the team doctor sent her to me to begin treatment. Her baseline testing was terrible; her balance was way off, she was dizzy, she had a bad headache, and she was still throwing up. I immediately treated her with laser therapy to the cranium and vagus nerve. I did manual muscle release for her head and neck. Then we started working on her balance and doing gaze stabilization exercises. I also put her on a nutrition and supplements protocol and started the leaky gut prevention protocol. By the end of our first session, her nausea had subsided quite a bit and her headache was better. We continued with daily sessions for the next week, and then went to three times a week for the next two weeks. She was back on the exercise bike on day five after the concussion. By the end of three weeks, she was cleared to play again, with no concerns about second impact syndrome. That season turned out to be her best ever both on the field and in the classroom.

Conclusion

An Inside-Out Life

If all you have is a hammer, everything looks like a nail. Patients need practitioners who have efficient toolboxes that can individualize treatment.

The patient is the evidence.

In every chapter of this book, I've rejected the idea of treating just the symptoms of a health issue and instead focused on finding and treating the true source of the problem. The treatment is almost always something that helps the problem from the inside out using a natural, functional approach instead of drugs or surgery.

The rent for your health is due every day. As the great inspirational speaker Jim Rohm says, "Take care of your body. It's the only place you have to live."

THE DASH

You know how on your tombstone it says the year you were born and the year you died, with a dash in between? The dash is the important part. What did you do to fill the years of that dash? Were you a good person, a good family member, a good friend? Did you help people? I want my dash to be filled with people who are better in every way because I was able to help them improve their health.

Originally I went back to school to learn how to help the patients in front of me. Then I took another step and began to help them at seminars. Now I've written this book because I want as many people as possible to know that better health is within their reach.

LIVING THE THERAPEUTIC LIFE

Every year, we spend $765 million on treating lower back pain. Some 96 percent of every dollar spent on Medicare is for treating a chronic disease; that number is 83 percent for Medicaid. Much of that money is spent unnecessarily on health problems that could have been prevented and could be treated with simple lifestyle and dietary changes.

In this book I hope I've shown you how to have a therapeutic lifestyle from the inside out. I hope I've shown you the importance of moving well. Today, sitting is the new smoking. Just in the past few years, we've seen a lot of research in the medical journals warning about the dangers of a sedentary life. If you sit most of the day for your work, even an hour-long session at the gym on the way home may not be enough to overcome the damage. And if you sit all day at work and then sit in front of the TV all evening, the damage could be cutting years off your life expectancy.

Why don't people exercise more? Because their bodies hurt, usually as a result of uncorrected damage and poor motion that leads to injury, reinjury, and chronic pain. When they first come to see me, many of my patients have serious limitations to their movements. Some can barely walk; others can't raise their arms above their heads or pick up a toddler. Before I can get them to make exercise a regular part of their day, I have to help them learn to move well again. That's more than just treating the outward problem. We have to work from the inside out by changing their lifestyles, decreasing their stress, detoxifying them, supplementing what's missing from their nutrition, and improving their diet.

The therapeutic lifestyle is a commitment to your own health. It's not always easy to stick with it. That's OK. If you fall off the horse, it's not the end of the world—it's a chance to start again. Remember, this is a lifestyle, not a race that's over when you cross the finish line. When I start working with a new patient, we set some short- and long-term goals. The short-term goal is just to get there— to fix the problem and get on the path to better health. The long-term goal is the harder goal. It's to stay there, to value it, and to enjoy it.

To help my patients stick with long-term goals, I educate them. I explain, as often as it takes, why we're doing what we're doing, what we hope to accomplish, and how that will help. I hope that what you've learned from this book will lead you to take action. Knowledge plus action equals power—and that power is your health. As long as you have your health, you have the ability to do whatever you want. I often think about what Norman Cousins, an early leader in holistic health, once said: "The tragedy of life is not death but what we let die inside of us while we live." Never let your zest for health die.

I WANT TO HELP

My wick burns 24-7, 365. I'm always available to help you restore your health. Call me at my office at 914-287-6464, email me at info@drrobertsilverman.com, contact me through my website at drrobertsilverman.com, or reach me through:

facebook.com/drrobertsilverman

@yoursportsdoc

@nychirocare

I'll help you light your candle, and together we'll move forward to vibrant good health.

About the Author

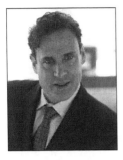

DR. ROBERT G. SILVERMAN graduated magna cum laude from the University of Bridgeport College of Chiropractic and has a Masters of Science in human nutrition. His extensive list of educational accomplishments includes designations as a certified nutrition specialist, certified clinical nutritionist and a certified sports nutritionist. Dr. Silverman is a diplomate with the American Clinical Board of Nutrition and the Chiropractic Board of Nutrition.

He is an internationally known speaker and author with a full-time private practice in White Plains, NY, where he specializes in the treatment of joint pain with innovative, science-based, nonsurgical approaches and functional medicine.

Dr. Silverman is also on the advisory board for the Functional Medicine University. He is a health contributor to Fox News Radio and has appeared on *Fox & Friends*, *Fox News*, *NBC News*, *CBS News*, *Wall Street Journal Live*, and *NewsMax TV*.

He was awarded the prestigious 2015 Sports Chiropractor of the Year by the ACA Sports Council.